WO 660

The AST Handbook of Transplant Infections

Disclaimer

This Document is provided for informational and general educational purposes only. This Document should not be used in place of professional medical advice and is not intended to be a substitute for consultation with or treatment by a medical professional. This Document is an educational tool designed only to enhance and support the treatment and education process. This Document should not be substituted for specific medical advice or instruction by a physician, nurse or pharmacist.

The AST Handbook of Transplant Infections

EDITED BY

Deepali Kumar MD MSc FRCPC

Transplant Infectious Diseases
University of Alberta
Edmonton
Canada

Atul Humar MD MSc FRCPC

Transplant Infections Diseases
University of Alberta
Edmonton
Canada

Associate Editors

Emily Blumberg MD
Marian G. Michaels MD, MPH
Kieren Marr MD

On behalf of The American Society of Transplantation
Infectious Diseases Community of Practice

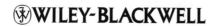

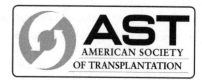

A John Wiley & Sons, Ltd., Publication

This edition first published 2011, © 2011 by Blackwell Publishing Ltd

Blackwell Publishing was acquired by John Wiley & Sons in February 2007. Blackwell's publishing program has been merged with Wiley's global Scientific, Technical and Medical business to form Wiley-Blackwell.

Registered office: John Wiley & Sons Ltd, The Atrium, Southern Gate, Chichester, West Sussex, PO19 8SQ, UK

Editorial offices: 9600 Garsington Road, Oxford, OX4 2DQ, UK
The Atrium, Southern Gate, Chichester, West Sussex, PO19 8SQ, UK
111 River Street, Hoboken, NJ 07030-5774, USA

For details of our global editorial offices, for customer services and for information about how to apply for permission to reuse the copyright material in this book please see our website at www.wiley.com/wiley-blackwell

Library of Congress Cataloging-in-Publication Data

The AST handbook of transplant infections / edited by Deepali Kumar, Atul Humar ; associate editors, Emily Blumberg, Marian Michaels, Kieren Marr ; on behalf of the American Society of Transplantation Infectious Diseases Community of Practice.
    p. ; cm.
    Handbook of transplant infections
    Includes bibliographical references and index.
    ISBN 978-0-470-65827-7 (pbk. : alk. paper) 1. Communicable diseases—Handbooks, manuals, etc. 2. Transplantation of organs, tissues, etc.—Complications—Handbooks, manuals, etc. I. Kumar, Deepali. II. Humar, Atul. III. American Society of Transplantation. Infectious Diseases Community of Practice. IV. Title: Handbook of transplant infections.
    [DNLM: 1. Transplants—adverse effects—Handbooks. 2. Bacterial Infections—therapy—Handbooks. 3. Mycoses—therapy—Handbooks. 4. Virus Diseases—therapy—Handbooks. WO 39]
    RC112.A88 2011
    616.9'8—dc22
                                                                                              2011002978

ISBN: 9780470658277

A catalogue record for this book is available from the British Library.

This book is published in the following electronic formats: ePDF 9781444397925; Wiley Online Library 9781444397949; ePub 9781444397932

Set in 9/12pt Meridien by MPS Limited, a Macmillan Company, Chennai, India
Printed and bound in Malaysia by Vivar Printing Sdn Bhd.

1 2011

Contents

List of Contributors

Upton D. Allen MBBS, MSc, FAAP, FRCPC, FRCP (UK)
Professor, Departments of
Paediatrics and Health Policy
Management and Evaluation
University of Toronto
Division Head, Infectious Diseases
The Hospital for Sick Children
Toronto, Canada

Lindsey R. Baden MD
Division of Infectious Disease
Brigham and Women's Hospital
Dana Farber Cancer Institute
Boston, MA, USA

Emily A. Blumberg MD
Professor of Medicine
Division of Infectious Diseases
University of Pennsylvania School of
Medicine
Philadelphia, PA, USA

Bartholomew Bono MD
Program Director, Infectious
Disease
Albert Einstein Healthcare Network
Philadelphia, PA, USA

Steven D. Burdette MD, FIDSA
Infectious Diseases Fellowship
Director & Associate Professor
of Medicine
Infectious Disease Advisor to Miami
Valley Hospital Transplant Program
WSU Boonshoft School of Medicine
Dayton, OH, USA

Nina M. Clark MD
Associate Professor
Department of Internal Medicine
University of Illinois at Chicago
Chicago, IL, USA

Lara Danziger-Isakov MD, MPH
Staff, Center for Pediatric Infectious
Diseases; Director for Pediatric Clinical
Research
The Children's Hospital at Cleveland
Clinic
Assistant Professor of Pediatrics
Cleveland Clinic Lerner College of
Medicine at CWRU
Cleveland, OH, USA

Karen Doucette MD, MSc (Epi), FRCPC
Associate Professor, Division of
Infectious Diseases
Education Director, Transplant
Infectious Diseases Fellowship
University of Alberta
Edmonton, AB, USA

Staci A. Fischer MD, FACP, FIDSA
Associate Professor of Medicine
The Warren Alpert Medical School of
Brown University
Director, Transplant Infectious Diseases
Rhode Island Hospital
Providence, RI, USA

Julia Garcia-Diaz MD, MS, FACP
Department of Infectious Diseases
Ochsner Clinic Foundation
New Orleans, LA, USA

Christian Garzoni MD
University Clinic for Infectious Disease
Bern University Hospital, Inselspital
Bern, Switzerland

Michael Green MD, MPH
Professor of Pediatrics, Surgery &
Clinical and Translational Science
University of Pittsburgh School of Medicine
Division of Infectious Diseases
Children's Hospital of Pittsburgh
Pittsburgh, PA, USA

Sarah P. Hammond MD
Instructor of Medicine
Harvard Medical School
Division of Infectious Diseases
Brigham and Women's Hospital
Boston, MA, USA

Lizbeth Hansen
Cleveland Clinic
Lerner College of Medicine at CWRU
Cleveland, OH, USA

Betsy Herold MD
Professor, Department of Pediatrics
(Infectious Diseases)
Professor, Department of Microbiology &
Immunology
Professor, Department of
Obstetrics & Gynecology and
Women's Health
Albert Einstein College of Medicine
New York
NY, USA

Hans H. Hirsch MD, MSc, FMH (Inf Diseases), FMH (Internal Medicine), FAMH (Medical Microbiology)
Acting Director, Institute for Medical
Microbiology
Department of Biomedicine
University of Basel, and
Attending Physician,
Division of Infectious Diseases &
Hospital Epidemiology
University Hospital Basel
Basel, Switzerland

S.M. Hosseini-Mogaddham
Urology and Nephrology Research
Center (UNRC)
Shahid Beheshti University
Tehran, Iran

Jennifer Hsu MD
Division of Infectious Diseases
Department of Medicine
University of Wisconsin School of
Medicine and Public Health
Madison, WI, USA

Robert Huang MD
Department of Medicine
Division of Infectious Diseases
University of California at San Diego
La Jolla, CA, USA

Abhinav Humar MD
Professor, Department of Surgery
Clinical Director, Starzl Transplant
Institute
University of Pittsburgh
Pittsburgh, PA, USA

Shirish Huprikar MD
Director, Transplant Infectious Diseases
Program
Associate Professor, Department of
Medicine
Mount Sinai School of Medicine
New York, NY, USA

Shahid Husain MD, MS
Assistant Professor of Medicine
Director, Transplant Infectious
Diseases
Division of Infectious Diseases and
Multi-organ Transplantation
University Health Network/University
of Toronto
Toronto, Canada

Michael G. Ison MD MS
Assistant Professor, Divisions of
Infectious Diseases and Organ
Transplantation
Northwestern University Feinberg
School of Medicine
Medical Director, Transplant &
Immunocompromised Host
Infectious Diseases Service
Northwestern University
Comprehensive Transplant Center
Chicago, IL, USA

Kathleen Julian MD
Assistant Professor of Medicine
Division of Infectious Diseases
Penn State Hershey Medical Center
Hershey, PA, USA

Daniel Kaul MD
Director, Transplant ID Service
Division of Infectious Disease
University of Michigan Medical School
Ann Arbor, MI USA

Camille Nelson Kotton MD
Clinical Director, Transplant and
Immunocompromised Host Infectious
Diseases
Infectious Diseases Division
Massachusetts General Hospital and
Assistant Professor
Harvard Medical School
Harvard University
Boston, MA, USA

Lynne Lewis RN, MS, CPNP
Coordinator, Division of Pediatric
Infectious Diseases
Section on Immunocompromised Hosts
Children's Hospital Boston
Boston, MA, USA

Rebecca P. Madan MD, MSc
Assistant Professor
Division of Pediatric Infectious Diseases
Albert Einstein College of Medicine
New York, NY, USA

Oriol Manuel MD
Infectious Diseases Service and
Transplantation Center
University Hospital Center (CHUV) and
University of Lausanne
Lausanne, Switzerland

Francisco M. Marty MD
Division of Infectious Disease
Brigham and Women's Hospital
Boston, MA, USA

Sanjay R. Mehta MD, DTM&H
Assistant Clinical Professor of Medicine
Division of Infectious Diseases
University of California
San Diego, CA, USA

Aneesh K. Mehta MD
Assistant Professor of Medicine
Assistant Director of Transplant
Infectious Diseases
Division of Infectious Diseases
Emory University School of Medicine
Atlanta, GA, USA

Marian G. Michaels MD, MPH
Professor of Pediatrics and Surgery
University of Pittsburgh School of
Medicine
Children's Hospital of Pittsburgh of
UPMC
Division of Pediatric Infectious
Diseases
Pittsburgh, PA, USA

**Michele I. Morris MD, FACP,
FIDSA**
Clinical Chief, Division of Infectious
Diseases
Director, Immunocompromised Host
Section
Associate Professor of Clinical Medicine
University of Miami Miller School of
Medicine
Miami, FL, USA

**Sherif Beniameen Mossad MD,
FACP, FIDSA**
Staff Department of Infectious Diseases
Section Head of Transplant Infectious
Diseases
Medicine Institute and Transplant
Center
Associate Professor of Medicine
CCLCM of CWRU Cleveland
OH, USA

Nicolas J. Mueller MD
Senior Attending Physician
Division of Infectious Diseases and
Hospital Epidemiology
University Hospital Zurich
Zurich, Switzerland

**Elizabeth A. Neuner PharmD,
BCPS**
Infectious Diseases Clinical Specialist
Department of Pharmacy
Cleveland Clinic
Cleveland, OH, USA

Raymund R. Razonable MD
Associate Professor of Medicine
Director, Transplant Infectious
Diseases
Associate Chair for Faculty
Development and Diversity
Division of Infectious Diseases
College of Medicine
Mayo Clinic Rochester, MN, USA

Gail Elizabeth Reid MD, BA
Assistant Professor of Medicine
Division of Infectious Diseases
Deparment of Medicine
University of Illinois
Chicago Medical Center
Chicago, IL, USA

Nasia Safdar MD, PhD
Hospital Epidemiologist
UWHC Section of Infectious
Diseases
Department of Medicine and Infection
Control
University of Wisconsin-Madison
School of Medicine and Public
Health
and Wm S Middleton VA Center
Madison, WI, USA

Tanvi Sharma MD
Instructor in Pediatrics, Assistant in
Medicine
Division of Pediatric Infectious Diseases
Children's Hospital Boston and Harvard
Medical School
Boston, MA, USA

Shmuel Shoham MD, FACP
Scientific Director, MedStar Clinical
Research Center and
Director, Transplant Infectious Diseases
Washington Hospital Center
Washington, DC, USA

Germana L.M. Silva MD
Resident, Medical College of Wisconsin
Department of Anesthesiology
Milwaukee, WI, USA

Valentina Stosor MD
Associate Professor
Division of Infectious Diseases
Chicago, IL, USA

Christian van Delden MD
Head, Immunocompromised Host
Program
Service of Infectious Diseases
Department of Medical Specialties
University Hospital
Geneva, Switzerland

Marissa B. Wilck MD
Division of Infectious Disease
Brigham and Women's Hospital
Dana Farber Cancer Institute
Boston, MA, USA

Preface

Transplantation is a complex, multidisciplinary specialty. Modern immunosuppressive therapy has improved patient and graft outcome. However, this places transplant patients at risk for a variety of infectious complications. Advances in transplant infectious diseases such as molecular diagnostics and novel therapeutics, coupled with the changing epidemiology of infectious agents, have greatly increased the complexity surrounding appropriate prevention and management of infections in these patients.

This is the first edition of the *AST Handbook of Transplant Infections*. It offers practical guidance on both common and unusual issues encountered in both solid organ and hematopoietic stem cell transplant patients. The handbook offers a practical approach to specific clinical syndromes after transplantation, as well as diagnosis, prevention and therapy of specific infections. We also address scenarios related to the prevention of donor-derived infections, common drug interactions, and other issues specifically related to the transplant patient.

The book does not go through comprehensive dosing or spectrum of activity of commonly used antimicrobials. It is assumed that the reader has some general knowledge of antimicrobials, their overall spectrum of coverage and dose adjustments in renal failure.

The handbook will be updated regularly. This book is endorsed by the American Society of Transplantation (AST). We acknowledge the members of the AST Infectious Diseases Community of Practice, whose members conceived the idea, and wrote and reviewed the chapters. In addition, we thank the members of the AST Pharmacy Community of Practice for reviewing selected sections.

We hope that you will find the handbook useful in your daily clinical practice.

Deepali Kumar & Atul Humar
Edmonton

Acknowledgements

We would like to gratefully acknowledge the following individuals who contributed as reviewers to the 2011 edition of the handbook:

Emily Blumberg, Barrett R. Crowther, Lara Danziger-Isakov, Steven Gabardi, Shirish Huprikar, Michael Ison, Sarah Jones, Zakiyah Kadry, Tsing Yi Koh-Pham, Camille Kotton, Oriol Manuel, Kieren Marr, Marian Michaels, Raymund Razonable, Christin Rogers, Nina Singh, Eric M. Tichy, and Nicole A. Weimert.

We would also like to thank the AST Pharmacy Community of Practice for their review of the handbook.

Acknowledgements

PART I
General Issues and Infectious Syndromes

1 Timeline of Infections After Organ Transplant

Christian van Delden

Time post-transplant	0–1 month	1–6 months	>6 months
Type of infection	Nosocomial infections: pneumonia, catheter-related, UTI Post-surgical infections: wound, anastomotic leaks, abscesses Donor-derived infections	Opportunistic infections Reactivation of recipient or donor latent infections (prophylaxis may shift further)	Community-acquired infections In the absence of prophylaxis: reactivation of latent infections during intense immunosuppression for acute graft rejection
Bacterial	*C. difficile* colitis Antimicrobial resistant bacteria (MRSA, VRE, ESBL, MDR Gram-negative rods) Post-surgical infections (infected biliomas in liver transplant, pneumonia in lung transplant, UTI in renal transplant)	*Listeria, Nocardia* (if no TMP/SMX) *Mycobacterium tuberculosis, Legionella*	Ongoing risk for *Listeria, Nocardia, M. tuberculosis, Legionella* if ongoing intense immunosuppression Graft-related infections (cholangitis in liver, pneumonia in lung, UTI in kidney) Community-acquired pneumonia pathogens
Viral	In the absence of anti-herpesvirus prophylaxis: HSV Donor-derived: LCMV, rhabdovirus, West Nile virus, HIV	BK nephropathy (kidney), HCV reactivation (liver), adenovirus, respiratory viruses CMV, EBV, HSV, VZV (after discontinuation of prophylaxis)	Late onset CMV (post-prophylaxis), EBV-related PTLD, recurrent HSV, VZV, HCV progression, JC polyomavirus (PML) Respiratory viruses, enteric viruses, West Nile virus
Fungal	*Candida* spp. Early *Aspergillus* only in some settings	*Cryptococcus, Aspergillus,* atypical molds, *Zygomycetes* sp. *Pneumocystis* only if no prophylaxis	During intense immunosuppression in the absence of antifungal prophylaxis: *Aspergillus*, atypical molds, Zygomycetes species Geographically restricted endemic fungi
Parasitic	Uncommon	*Toxoplasma, Strongyloides, Trypanosoma, Leishmania*	Ongoing risk if intense immunosuppression

CMV, cytomegalovirus; EBV, Epstein—Barr virus; ESBL, extended spectrum beta-lactamase; HCV, hepatitis C virus; HIV, human immunodeficiency virus; HSV, herpes simplex virus; LCMV, lymphocytic choriomeningitis virus; MDR, multi-drug-resistant; MRSA, methicillin-resistant *Staphylococcus aureus*; PML, progressive multifocal leukoencephalopathy; PTLD, post-transplant lymphoproliferative disorder; SMX, sulfamethoxazole; TMP, trimethoprim; UTI, urinary tract infection; VRE, vancomycin-resistant enterococci; VZV, varicella zoster virus.

The AST Handbook of Transplant Infections, 1st edition. Edited by D. Kumar & A. Humar. © 2011 Blackwell Publishing Ltd.

2 Timeline of Infections After Hematopoietic Stem Cell Transplant

Sarah P. Hammond & Francisco M. Marty

Time period	Pre-engraftment (day 0 to days 10–30*)	Early post-engraftment (up to day 100)	Mid post-engraftment (up to 1 year)	Late post-engraftment (after 1 year)
Infection risk factors	Neutropenia Mucositis Venous catheters	Immunosuppression (aGVHD) Venous catheters	Immunosuppression (cGVHD)	Immunosuppression (cGVHD)
Type of infection	Chemotherapy-associated and nosocomial infections	Opportunistic infections	Opportunistic and community infections	Community-acquired infections
Bacterial	Gram-positive cocci			
	Gram-negative rods*			
		Encapsulated bacteria		
		Listeria/Salmonella/Nocardia		
Viral	BK virus hemorrhagic cystitis		VZV**	
	HSV		EBV/PTLD**	
		CMV*		
		HHV-6/adenovirus reactivation**		HBV reactivation**
		Respiratory and enteric viral infections (influenza, RSV, parainfluenza, norovirus)		
Fungal	Candida*			
	Aspergillus	Aspergillus and other molds (mucorales)†		
		Pneumocystis jirovecii pneumonia		
Parasitic	Strongyloides hyperinfection**			
		Toxoplasma reactivation**		

| High risk | Moderate risk | Low risk | High risk, but prophylaxis typically given |

aGVHD, acute graft-versus-host disease; cGVHD, chronic GVHD; CMV, cytomegalovirus; EBV, Epstein–Barr virus; HBV, hepatitis B virus; HSV, herpes simplex virus; PTLD, post-transplant lymphoproliferative disorder; VZV, varicella zoster virus.

*Some centers mitigate this risk with prophylaxis.

**In previously exposed recipients.

†High risk in those with severe GVHD.

Source: Marty FM, Baden LR (2008). Infection in the Hematopoetic Stem Cell Transplant Recipient. In: Soiffer RJ, ed. *Hematopoietic Stem Cell Transplantation.* Totowa, NJ, USA: Humana Press, 421–448.

The AST Handbook of Transplant Infections, 1st edition. Edited by D. Kumar & A. Humar. © 2011 Blackwell Publishing Ltd.

3 Immune Reconstitution After Myeloablative Stem Cell Transplant

Sarah P. Hammond & Francisco M. Marty

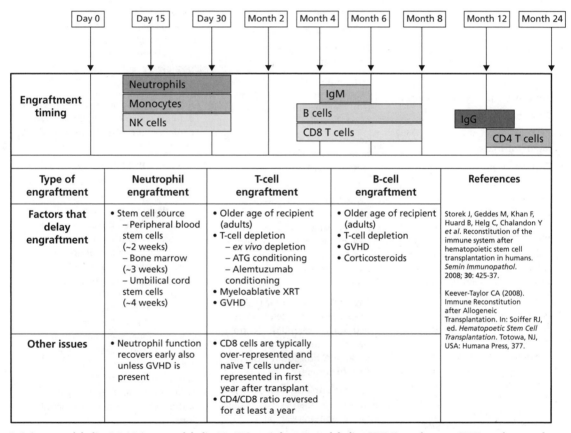

Type of engraftment	Neutrophil engraftment	T-cell engraftment	B-cell engraftment	References

Factors that delay engraftment	• Stem cell source
	  – Peripheral blood stem cells (~2 weeks)
	  – Bone marrow (~3 weeks)
	  – Umbilical cord stem cells (~4 weeks)
		• Older age of recipient (adults)
		• T-cell depletion
		  – *ex vivo* depletion
		  – ATG conditioning
		  – Alemtuzumab conditioning
		• Myeloablative XRT
		• GVHD
			• Older age of recipient (adults)
			• T-cell depletion
			• GVHD
			• Corticosteroids
				Storek J, Geddes M, Khan F, Huard B, Helg C, Chalandon Y et al. Reconstitution of the immune system after hematopoietic stem cell transplantation in humans. *Semin Immunopathol.* 2008; **30**: 425-37.
				
				Keever-Taylor CA (2008). Immune Reconstitution after Allogeneic Transplantation. In: Soiffer RJ, ed. *Hematopoetic Stem Cell Transplantation.* Totowa, NJ, USA: Humana Press, 377.

Other issues	• Neutrophil function recovers early also unless GVHD is present	• CD8 cells are typically over-represented and naïve T cells under-represented in first year after transplant • CD4/CD8 ratio reversed for at least a year		

IgG, immunoglobulin G; IgM, immunoglobulin M; ATG, anti-thymocyte globulin ; XRT, X-ray therapy; GVHD, graft-versus-host disease.

The AST Handbook of Transplant Infections, 1st edition. Edited by D. Kumar & A. Humar. © 2011 Blackwell Publishing Ltd.

4 Pre-transplant Infectious Disease Evaluation of the Organ Transplant Candidate

Staci A. Fischer

Routine screening	Optional testing (if clinically indicated only)	Organ-specific considerations
• CMV antibody • EBV antibody • HIV antibody • Hepatitis C antibody • Hepatitis B surface antigen and antibody; hepatitis B core antibody • Rapid plasma reagin • PPD or interferon-release assay for latent tuberculosis • *Toxoplasma* antibody (in heart transplant candidates) • Recipients should be screened for protective antibody to vaccine-preventable viral infections, particularly varicella, measles and mumps. Those without IgG antibody should be vaccinated pre-transplant if not already on immunosuppressive therapy • A thorough history should be completed to identify potential exposures to infections with a latent or chronic phase which could reactivate on immunosuppressive therapy. Such infections include *Mycobacterium tuberculosis*, endemic fungi such as *Coccidioides*, and *Strongyloides* (see 'Optional testing' column) • Should an infection be identified in the screening of the potential organ transplant recipient, consultation with an infectious	• HSV antibody • HTLV-I/II antibody • *Toxoplasma* antibody (in non-heart transplant candidates) • *Trypanosoma cruzi* antibody in recipients from endemic areas (e.g. Mexico, Central America, South America) • *Coccidioides* antibody in recipients from endemic areas (e.g. southwestern USA, Mexico, Central America, South America) • *Histoplasma* antibody in recipients from endemic areas (e.g. Ohio and Mississippi river valleys in the USA, other river valleys in North and Central America, Eastern and Southern Europe, Africa and Australia) • *Strongyloides* antibody in recipients from endemic areas (e.g. Appalachian USA, Central America, South America, sub-Saharan Africa, South-east Asia, Eastern Europe) • *Brucella* serology in recipients from endemic areas (e.g. Middle East, Mediterranean basin, eastern Europe, Asia, Africa, Central and South America). Ingestion of unpasteurized milk or chesses from endemic areas is a risk factor for infection	Patients with end-stage organ disease are susceptible to certain infections which should be diagnosed and treated prior to transplantation if at all possible. Specific considerations include the following: • *Kidney* – hemodialysis catheter-related bloodstream infections, peritonitis in peritoneal dialysis patients, hepatitis B, hepatitis C, complicated UTIs • *Pancreas* – wounds and osteomyelitis related to diabetic neuropathy • *Heart* – infection of ventricular assist devices (localized drive line infections or bloodstream infections mimicking endocarditis) should be aggressively treated but do not preclude transplantation. Chagas disease (trypanosomiasis) should be ruled out in the patient from an endemic area with dilated cardiomyopathy. Toxoplasmosis is a particular concern in cardiac transplantation, in which donor transmission can occur in the seronegative recipient of a seropositive heart, resulting in acute myocarditis or disseminated infection • *Liver* – hepatitis B, hepatitis C, cholangitis, spontaneous bacterial peritonitis, intravenous catheter-related infections, including candidemia

(Continued)

The AST Handbook of Transplant Infections, 1st edition. Edited by D. Kumar & A. Humar. © 2011 Blackwell Publishing Ltd.

Routine screening	Optional testing (if clinically indicated only)	Organ-specific considerations
disease specialist may be indicated to guide pre-transplant treatment, timing of transplantation when delay is possible, and/or post-transplant monitoring	• West Nile Virus serology • Human herpes virus-8 (HHV-8) serology • BK virus serology (kidney transplantation)	• *Lung* – sputum cultures to determine colonizing bacteria, mycobacteria and fungi should guide perioperative anti-microbial choices

CMV, cytomegalovirus; EBV, Epstein–Barr virus; HSV, herpes simplex virus; HTLV, human T-cell lymphotrophic virus; IgG, immunoglobulin G; PPD, purified protein derivative; UTI, urinary tract infection.

References: [1] *Am J Transplantation* 2009; 9(s4): S7 (updated guidelines on screening donors and recipients); [2] *Clin Infect Dis* 2002; 35: 1513 (detailed discussion of screening of recipients prior to transplantation); [3] *Clin Infect Dis* 1997; 24: 18; [4] www.cdc.gov/travel/yellowbook/2010 (updated information on travel-related infections with details on areas of endemicity for the pathogens noted above).

5 Pre-transplant Infectious Disease Evaluation of the Hematopoietic Stem Cell Transplant Candidate

Staci A. Fischer

Routine screening of all recipients	Optional testing (if clinically indicated only)	Comments
• CMV • EBV antibody • HIV antibody, NAT • Hepatitis C antibody, NAT • Hepatitis B surface antigen and antibody; hepatitis B core antibody • HSV-1 and 2 antibody • Rapid plasma reagin • Varicella zoster virus IgG • PPD testing (the role of interferon-release assays for detection of latent tuberculosis in the potential HSCT recipient is currently unclear)	• Hepatitis B NAT • HTLV-I/II antibodies • West Nile virus NAT • *Toxoplasma* IgG antibody • *Trypanosoma cruzi* antibody in donors from endemic areas (e.g. Mexico, Central America, South America) • *Strongyloides* antibody in recipients from endemic areas (e.g., Appalachian USA, Central America, South America, sub-Saharan Africa, South-east Asia, eastern Europe) • *Coccidioides* antibody in recipients from endemic areas (e.g. south-western USA, Mexico, Central America, South America) • *Histoplasma* antibody in recipients from endemic areas (e.g. Ohio and Mississippi river valleys in the USA, other river valleys in North and Central America, eastern and southern Europe, Africa and Australia) • *Brucella* serology in recipients from endemic areas (e.g. Middle East, Mediterranean basin, eastern Europe, Asia, Africa, Central and South America). Ingestion of unpasteurized milk or cheeses from endemic areas is a risk factor for infection	A detailed exposure (travel and residence) history should be obtained, with testing guided as in the 'Optional testing' column **Resources** *MMWR* 2000; 49(RR10): 1–128 (comprehensive guidelines for prevention of infection in HSCT) www.fda.gov/BiologicsBloodVaccines/SafetyAvailability/TissueSafety – *Testing HCT/P Donors for Relevant Communicable Disease Agents and Diseases* (updated guidelines for testing blood and HSCT donors for infections including information on specific FDA-approved assays) www.aabb.org/Content/Blood_Donor_History_Questionnaires/HPC-Donor_History_Questionnaire (updated questionnaire for potential blood and HSCT donors, including algorithms for inclusion/exclusion criteria based on results of infection testing) www.advanceweb.com/MLP (ADVANCE for Medical Laboratory Professionals, 2007 – blood donor screening process and infectious disease testing using molecular methods) www.cdc.gov/travel/yellowbook/2010 (Centers for Disease Control and Prevention – updated information on travel-related infections with details on areas of endemicity for the pathogens noted above)

CMV, cytomegalovirus; EBV, Epstein–Barr virus; HIV, human immunodeficiency virus; HSCT, hematopoietic stem cell transplant; HCT/Ps, human cell, tissues and cellular and tissue-based products; HSV, herpes simplex virus; HTLV, human T-cell lymphotrophic virus; IgG, immunoglobulin G; NAT, nucleic acid testing; PPD, purified protein derivative.

Screening of HSCT recipients includes screening for active infection, which could worsen with conditioning regimens, and for latent infections, which could reactivate during therapy administered to combat graft-versus-host disease. The risk of infection is much greater in recipients of allogeneic transplants than in recipients of autologous transplants.

The AST Handbook of Transplant Infections, 1st edition. Edited by D. Kumar & A. Humar. © 2011 Blackwell Publishing Ltd.

6 Technical Complications after Organ Transplant and Associated Infections

Abhinav Humar

6.1 Anastomoses and potential technical complications associated with either a pancreas transplant or kidney transplant*

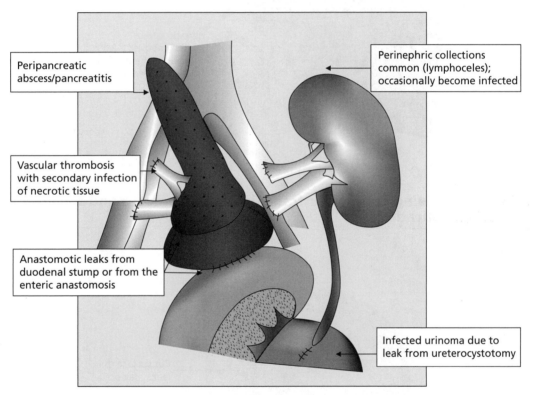

Peripancreatic abscess/pancreatitis

Perinephric collections common (lymphoceles); occasionally become infected

Vascular thrombosis with secondary infection of necrotic tissue

Anastomotic leaks from duodenal stump or from the enteric anastomosis

Infected urinoma due to leak from ureterocystotomy

*Only shows enteric drainage of the pancreas. Bladder drainage of pancreatic exocrine secretions is also possible.

The AST Handbook of Transplant Infections, 1st edition. Edited by D. Kumar & A. Humar. © 2011 Blackwell Publishing Ltd.

6.2 **Anastomoses and potential technical complications associated with liver transplantation**

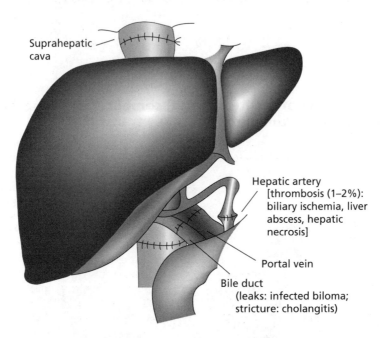

Suprahepatic cava

Hepatic artery [thrombosis (1–2%): biliary ischemia, liver abscess, hepatic necrosis]

Portal vein

Bile duct (leaks: infected biloma; stricture: cholangitis)

6.3 **Right lobe living donor liver transplant: anastomoses and selected technical complications**

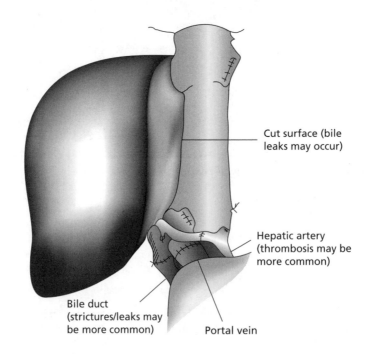

Cut surface (bile leaks may occur)

Hepatic artery (thrombosis may be more common)

Bile duct (strictures/leaks may be more common)

Portal vein

7 Evaluation and Initial Treatment of Infectious Complications Among Organ Transplant Recipients

Kathleen Julian

Site of infection		
Predominant pathogens	Diagnostic investigations	Initial empirical treatment in adult patients

GENERAL

Fever with no clear focus

Early post-transplant (< 1 month): infections at site of transplant (abscess), catheter-related or endovascular infections. Also consider donor-derived infections e.g. West Nile Virus, LCMV	Multiple blood cultures, urine culture, urinalysis with microscopy, CXR, CMV PCR/antigenemia	*Early post-transplant:* start empiric broad-spectrum antibiotics (e.g. piperacillin-tazobactam 3.375g IV q6h) after all cultures have been taken
Late post-transplant (> 1 month): broad differential: viral – CMV, HHV6, EBV(PTLD), adenovirus, respiratory viruses, parvovirus B19; bacterial – TB, MAC, *Nocardia*, occult abscess at transplant site; fungal – endemic mycoses, *Aspergillus*, PCP; parasitic – *Strongyloides*, toxoplasmosis, babesiosis	Image graft site, including vascular anastomosis (ultrasound or CT) If no diagnosis, consider full-body CT scan and EBV PCR Additional tests based on risk factors: nasopharyngeal swab for respiratory viruses PCR, viral PCRs on blood (e.g. parvovirus, adenovirus, HHV6, HIV, WNV); fungal and AFB blood cultures; urine/serum histoplasmosis & blastomycosis antigen; PPD or gamma interferon assay; syphilis screen, toxoplasmosis IgM or PCR (heart transplant); *Strongyloides* ELISA/stool for multiple O&P	*Late post-transplant:* if the patient is stable and not neutropenic, either start empiric antibiotics or consider withholding during initial work-up. If a clinical focus (e.g. pneumonia) is identified, see other sections of this table
Epidemiologic exposure may guide diagnosis: travel, animal, vector exposure; sexual exposure, etc. Non-infectious causes include rejection, drug fever, neoplasm.	If recent transplant, review donor information/contact OPO to see if other recipients also are developing similar presentations	

Septic shock syndrome without clinical focus

Broad range of infections, primarily bacterial and fungal, may cause acute septic shock	*Urgent* work-up as per under 'fever with no clear focus' to identify abscess or other underlying source	Immediately collect cultures and start broad-spectrum antibiotics: e.g. piperacillin-tazobactam 4.5g IV q6h *or* Meropenem 2g IV q8h + vancomycin 25–30mg IV loading dose × 1 then 15–20mg/kg IV q12h + ciprofloxacin 400 IV q8–12h

(Continued)

The AST Handbook of Transplant Infections, 1st edition. Edited by D. Kumar & A. Humar. © 2011 Blackwell Publishing Ltd.

(Continued)

Site of infection		
Predominant pathogens	**Diagnostic investigations**	**Initial empirical treatment in adult patients**
Potentially rapidly lethal causes of "septic shock" include bacteremia, vascular thrombosis of an intra-abdominal organ transplant, anastomic leak, cholangitis, necrotizing pancreatitis, toxic megacolon from *Clostridium difficile*, ischemic/necrotic bowel, bowel perforation including from CMV colitis, necrotizing fasciitis, toxic shock syndrome	Consider empiric discontinuation or replacement of central lines, and culturing catheter tips	If severe penicillin allergy, aztreonam 2 g IV q8h + vancomycin 25–30 mg IV loading dose × 1 then 15–20 mg/kg IV q8–12 + metronidazole 500 mg IV q6h ciprofloxacin 400 IV q8–12h Consider, in place of ciprofloxacin in above regimens, gentamicin 5–7 mg/kg IV q24 or colistimethate 2.5 mg/kg IV q12 in patients at risk for multi-drug resistant Gram negatives. Consider Echinocandin (e.g. caspofungin 70 mg IV loading dose × 1 then 50 mg IV q24h), especially if recent broad-spectrum antibiotics, TPN, or candida colonization Consider linezolid 600 mg IV q12h or daptomycin 6 mg/kg IV q24h (instead of vancomycin) if there is a recent history of VRE colonization/infection
Intravascular catheter-related infections Coagulase-negative staphylococci, *Staphylococcus aureus*, *Enterococcus* spp., enteric Gram-negative bacilli, *Pseudomonas* spp., *Candida* spp.	If drainage is present, swab entry site for culture Blood cultures × 2 (preferably one via catheter, one via peripheral venipuncture) Culture of catheter tip – aerobic and fungal cultures **Note**: If the patient has a single blood culture with a Gram-positive cocci or bacilli and is not on vancomycin or similar agent, collect an additional 2–3 blood cultures before initiating vancomycin (on the basis of four blood cultures collected prior to initiation of vancomycin, it may be easier later to distinguish contaminants from pathogens)	Vancomycin 15 mg/kg IV q12h + Gram-negative bacilli coverage (e.g. cefepime 2 g IV q12h *or* meropenem 1–2 g IV q8h *or* piperacillin-tazobactam 3.375 g IV q6h) [If severe penicillin allergy, then ciprofloxacin 400 mg IV q12h or aztreonam 2 g IV q8h for Gram-negative coverage] Consider antibiotic lock therapy to salvage lines in stable patients infected with organisms of low virulence (primarily, coagulase-negative staphylococci). Remove central catheters for most other organisms
CENTRAL NERVOUS SYSTEM **Central nervous system: acute meningitis/meningoencephalitis** Bacterial: *Listeria*, *Streptococcus pneumoniae*, *Neisseria meningitidis*, *Haemophilus influenzae*, Lyme disease, syphilis, *Rickettsia*	CT/MRI brain Lumbar puncture: opening pressure, CSF cell count and differential, protein, glucose, CSF bacterial, fungal, AFB	If suspect acute bacterial meningitis: ceftriaxone 2 g IV q12h + vancomycin loading dose of 25–30 mg/kg IV × 1, then 15–20 mg/kg IV q8–12h

Site of infection		
Predominant pathogens	Diagnostic investigations	Initial empirical treatment in adult patients
Viral: CMV, HSV, HHV6, VZV, WNV, enterovirus, measles, mumps Other: toxoplasmosis, *Strongyloides*, microabscesses due to disseminated fungal or bacterial infection Parameningeal infections (e.g. sinusitis, epidural infection) can cause a CSF pleocytosis WNV, LCMV, rabies, *Balamuthia*, *Naegleria* have been transmitted from organ donors Non-infectious: drug-induced (e.g. TMP/SMX, ATG), confusion and seizures caused by calcineurin inhibitors (PRES)	culture; cryptococcal CSF antigen; HSV PCR, enterovirus PCR, WNV PCR based on epidemiology. Consider other viral PCRs (CMV, HHV6, VZV). Keep additional tube of CSF for future studies. Cryptococcal serum antigen, CMV PCR or antigenemia Consider VDRL/FT-ABS on CSF; Lyme CSF EIA/PCR (with concurrent Lyme serum EIA); WNV serum IgM/IgG EIA and CSF IgM EIA. Consider leptospirosis IgM EIA, Rocky Mountain Spotted Fever IFA/ELISA, ehrlichiosis IFA/ELISA If recent transplant, review donor information/contact OPO to see if other recipients also are developing similar presentations	Consider adding ampicillin (for *Listeria*) 2 g IV q4h (especially if not on TMP/SMX prophylaxis) If CSF has lymphocytic pleocytosis: • Consider ganciclovir 5 mg/kg IV q12h, especially if encephalopathic • Consider lipid amphotericin product 5 mg/kg/day while awaiting results of cryptococcal testing • Consider doxycycline 100 mg IV q12h (loading dose 200 mg) for rickettsiae, including Rocky Mountain Spotted Fever in patients during tick season in endemic regions.
Meningitis: subacute, chronic Bacterial: *Mycobacterium tuberculosis*, Lyme, syphilis, *Brucella*, *Nocardia* Fungal: *Cryptococcus, Coccidioides immitis, Histoplasma capsulatum, Candida* and other fungi Other: toxoplasmosis, CNS PTLD	Head CT; consider also brain MRI (for other parameningeal processes, also consider spine MRI) Lumbar puncture: as above per acute meningitis, VDRL, TB PCR and AFB culture (large volume needed), Nocardia culture, cytology – keep additional tube of CSF for future studies PPD or interferon gamma assay, RPR (blood), Cryptococcal serum antigen Consider histoplasmosis antigen in CSF, coccidiomycosis complement fixation (CF) antibody in CSF; urine/serum histoplasmosis and blastomycosis antigen; Consider Lyme CSF EIA/PCR and concurrent Lyme serum EIA. Consider *Brucella* agglutinating antibody assay, toxoplasmosis IgM/IgG and toxoplasmosis PCR (if previously toxoplasmosis R−, especially after heart transplantation) CT body to identify evidence of systemic disease	Empiric therapy depends on clinical situation and most likely diagnosis. Might include therapy for *Cryptococcus*, TB, or other

(Continued)

(Continued)

Predominant pathogens	Diagnostic investigations	Initial empirical treatment in adult patients
	Site of infection	

Focal brain disease (abscess or space-occupying lesion)

Bacterial: septic emboli/local invasion from other sites of infection (broad mix of Gram-positive, anaerobes, Gram-negative bacteria), Nocardia, TB, Actinomyces, Listeria	CT/MRI brain	If bacterial brain abscess suspected – meropenem 2 g IV q8h ± vancomycin 15–20mg/kg IV q8–12h
	If lumbar puncture is safe, consider CSF studies as above plus EBV PCR and galactomannan antigen in CSF	Consider voriconazole 6 mg/kg IV q12h × 2 doses, then 4 mg/kg IV q12h or lipid amphotericin product 5–10mg/kg IV q24
Fungal: *Aspergillus*, zygomycetes, *Cryptococcus* and other	Consider CT body, echocardiogram to identify additional lesions (potentially more accessible to biopsy)	
Other: CNS PTLD, *Toxoplasma gondii*, neurocysticercosis	EBV PCR	
Non-infectious: other malignancy (primary or metastatic)	Consider toxoplasmosis serum IgM/IgG and PCR; serum cryptococcal antigen, serum galactomannan, histoplasmosis urinary antigen, blastomycosis urinary antigen. Consider cysticercosis serology, PPD or interferon gamma assay	
	Aspiration or biopsy under stereotactic CT guidance for aerobic, anaerobic, fungal, AFB, nocardia culture, Aspergillus PCR, TB PCR, and histopathology	

Progressive dementia

JC virus (progressive multifocal leukoencephalopathy); prion diseases; consider other causes of subacute/chronic meningoencephalitis listed above	MRI brain	Depends on etiology
	Consider CSF studies above, with addition of JC virus PCR of CSF	

RESPIRATORY
Pharyngitis, tonsillitis

Streptococcus pyogenes (group A), EBV (including PTLD), adenovirus, respiratory viruses	Swab of pharynx for streptococcal antigen (rapid) test or culture	Penicillin VK 250 mg PO QID for streptococcal pharyngitis *or* Azithromycin 500 mg PO on day 1, then 250 mg daily
	NP swab for respiratory virus PCR	
	EBV PCR	Oseltamivir 75 mg PO BID if influenza is suspected

Sinusitis: community-acquired

Streptococcus pneumoniae, *Haemophilus influenzae*, *Moraxella catarrhalis*, respiratory viruses	Red flags warranting urgent imaging/ENT evaluation: visual or neurologic involvement, prominent headache	Amoxicillin-clavulanate 875 mg PO BID *or* Levofloxacin 500 mg PO daily *or* Azithromycin 500 mg PO on day 1, then 250 mg PO
In CF lung transplant recipients, also *Pseudomonas*, *B. cepacia*	If there is no improvement after 48 h of decongestants and empirical antibiotic therapy or if patient has any red	

Site of infection		
Predominant pathogens	Diagnostic investigations	Initial empirical treatment in adult patients
Fungal: *Aspergillus* spp., zygomycetes	flags noted above, CT sinuses + ENT consult for aspiration of sinuses/biopsy	
	Consider serum galactomannan assay	
Sinusitis: nosocomial		
Aerobic/facultative, Gram-negative bacilli, *Staphylococcus aureus*, *Aspergillus* spp., Zygomycetes	CT sinuses ENT evaluation for endoscopy /sinus aspiration / biopsy	Piperacillin-tazobactam 4.5 g IV q6h *or* Cefepime 2 g IV q12h *or* Meropenem 1–2 g IV q8h
Pneumonia (excluding lung transplant)[a]		
Community-acquired: *Streptococcus pneumoniae*, *Haemophilus influenzae*, *Legionella* spp., *Moraxella catarrhalis*, *Mycoplasma pneumoniae*, *Chlamydia pneumonia*, respiratory viruses	CXR, CT chest Sputum/tracheal aspirate – bacterial, viral, Nocardia, fungal, AFB cultures, PCP stain, respiratory virus PCR (NP swab)	For community-acquired (no recent hospitalizations and post-transplant > 6 months) pneumonia not requiring ICU admission: a respiratory fluoroquinolone (e.g. moxifloxacin 400 mg) PO/IV daily or levofloxacin 750 mg PO/IV daily) *or* ceftriaxone 2 g IV daily + azithromycin 500 mg PO/ IV daily
Nosocomial: other Gram-negative bacilli (*Escherichia coli*, *Klebsiella pneumoniae*, *Pseudomonas aeruginosa*, *Acinetobacter* spp.), *Staphylococcus aureus* (including MRSA)	CMV PCR (or antigenemia), *Legionella* urine antigen Consider serum *Cryptococcus* antigen, serum galactomannan, urine/serum histoplasmosis and blastomycosis antigens	If possibility of influenza, add oseltamivir 75–150 mg PO BID For more severe or if nosocomial pneumonia: cefepime 2 g IV q8h–q12h *or* piperacillin-tazobactam 4.5 g IV q6h *or*
Opportunistic: fungal – *Aspergillus*, PCP, *Cryptococcus*, endemic fungi, zygomycetes, others; viral – CMV, HSV, VZV, adenovirus, others; bacterial – TB, other mycobacteria, *Nocardia*; parasitic – *Strongyloides*, toxoplasmosis	Low threshold for BAL: tests as above. Also consider BAL galactomannan, Nocardia culture or PCR assays for other pathogens (e.g. *Toxoplasma*, Nocardia), cytology	meropenem 2 g IV q8h + ciprofloxacin 400 mg IV q8–12h + agent for MRSA (vancomycin 25–30 mg IV loading dose × 1 then 15–20 mg/kg IV q12h *or* linezolid 600 IV q12h)
Non-infectious causes: multiple, including sirolimus pneumonitis, PTLD	If there is pleural effusion, consider thoracocentesis If there are nodular lesions and suspect fungal infection, pursue aggressive diagnostic testing (including BAL and CT-guided tissue biopsy or open-lung biopsy)	If no PCP prophylaxis, (especially within first year post-transplant), consider TMP/SMX (5 mg/kg of TMP component IV q6h) Consider (e.g., for nodular lesions) empiric voriconazole 6 mg/kg IV q12h × 1 day, then 4 mg/kg IV q12h
GASTROINTESTINAL/INTRA-ABDOMINAL **Oral cavity: stomatitis/mucositis (aphthous, ulcers)**		
HSV, CMV, *Candida* Sirolimus-related, idiopathic (aphthous) ulcers	Viral culture; HSV, DFA, PCR; consider CMV PCR/antigenemia	Valacyclovir 1 g PO BID

[a] For pneumonia in lung transplant, see chapter 11.

(Continued)

(Continued)

Site of infection		
Predominant pathogens	Diagnostic investigations	Initial empirical treatment in adult patients
Oral thrush		
Candida spp.	If atypical appearance, persistent, or relapsing, swab throat for fungal culture and sensitivity testing	Fluconazole 100-200 mg PO daily *or* Clotrimazole 10 mg troche five times per day *or* Nystatin suspension (100 000 U/mL) 4–6 mL four times daily, or 1–2 nystatin pastilles (200 000 U each) administered four times daily
Esophagitis		
HSV, CMV, *Candida* spp.	CMV PCR (or antigenemia) of blood Endoscopy and biopsy for viral culture, CMV PCR, histopathology	*Candida*: fluconazole 200-400 mg PO daily *or* caspofungin 50 mg IV q24 If suspect herpesvirus, consider valganciclovir 900 mg PO BID. If severe, consider ganciclovir 5 mg/kg IV q12h
Enteritis/colitis		
Bacteria: *Salmonella, Campylobacter, Listeria monocytogenes, Clostridium difficile* Viral: CMV, EBV (PTLD), enteric viruses (norovirus, adenovirus, rotavirus) Parasitic: *Strongyloides stercoralis, Entamoeba histolytica, Giardia lamblia* Other: small-bowel bacterial overgrowth, especially after liver transplant with Roux-en-Y reconstruction Non-infectious: include drug-induced (MMF, other), and other etiologies	Stool C&S, O&P; *C. difficile* toxin (if EIA, collect × 3; if cell culture assay, usually one sample is sufficient) CMV PCR/antigenemia Abdominal X-ray ± CT abdomen Consider *Vibrio* stool culture if has recently ingested seafood or visited seashore Consider testing of stool for enteric viruses (EIA, DFA, or PCR) Consider colonoscopy with biopsy for viral culture, CMV PCR, and histopathology. Also consider *Giardia* antigen (EIA) in stool, *Cryptosporidium* antigen (EIA) in stool, stool for modified AFB (cryptosporidia, isospora, cyclospora), chromotrope stain for microsporidia, serial O&P, Strongyloides ELISA	Depends on pathogen If recent antibiotics or severe illness, empiric *C. difficile* treatment (metronidazole or vancomycin, see chapter 30) Consider ciprofloxacin (400 IV q12h or 500–750 PO q12h) Consider empiric CMV treatment (ganciclovir 5 mg/kg IV q12h) while awaiting studies in high-risk persons with severe disease

(Continued)

Site of infection		
Predominant pathogens	Diagnostic investigations	Initial empirical treatment in adult patients
Intra-abdominal: peritoneum and peritoneal space		
Gram-negative bacilli (Enterobacteriaceae, *Pseudomonas aeruginosa*) *Enterococcus* spp., *Candida* spp., Anaerobic bacilli, (*Clostridium* spp., *Bacteroides* spp.)	Abdomen/pelvis CT Ultrasound of transplant vasculature (e.g. liver, pancreas, kidney transplants) Diagnostic sampling of peritoneal fluid/abscess. Check fluid bilirubin (liver transplant), creatinine (kidney transplant), or amylase (pancreas transplant)	Piperacillin-tazobactam 3.375 g IV q6h or meropenem 1–2 g IV q8h If unable to use β-lactams, vancomycin 15 mg/kg IV q12 + metronidazole 500 mg IV q6h + (ciprofloxacin 400 mg IV q12h *or* aztreonam 2 g IV q8h) ± *empiric antifungals*: fluconazole 400 mg IV/PO daily *or* echinocandin (e.g. caspofungin 70 mg IV load on day 1, then 50 mg IV daily) If VRE+, add linezolid 600 mg IV q12h *or* daptomycin 6 mg/kg IV q24h
Liver : hepatitis		
Viral: hepatitis A, B, C, E, CMV, HSV, EBV, VZV, HHV6, adenovirus Non-viral: usually as part of disseminated infection, e.g. fungal, mycobacterial Liver transplant: rejection, recurrent underlying disease, graft injury/ischemia Non-infectious: drug-induced	Image liver: ultrasound, CT, and/or MRI CMV PCR or antigenemia Depending on clinical situation, hepatitis A, B, C serology ± PCR If no diagnosis, consider other viral PCR such as adenovirus, HHV6, VZV, HSV, EBV, hepatitis E serology and PCR Liver biopsy for viral culture, CMV PCR, histopathology;	Depends on etiology
Liver abscess or cholangitis		
Gram-negative bacilli (Enterobacteriaceae, *Pseudomonas aeruginosa*, *Acinetobacter*), *Enterococcus*, *Candida* spp., *Staphylococcus aureus*, anaerobic bacilli	Image liver: ultrasound, CT, and/or MRI/ MRCP. For liver transplant, assess vessels, may need cholangiography	Piperacillin-tazobactam 3.375 g IV q6h *or* Vancomycin 15 mg/kg IV q12h + ciprofloxacin 400 IV q12 + metronidazole 500 mg IV q6h
In liver transplant, biliary stricture can lead to cholangitis, intrahepatic abscess formation. Hepatic artery thrombosis may also lead to recurrent hepatic abscesses	Aspiration of liver abscess under CT/ ultrasound guidance (prefer to delay antibiotics/antifungals until after aspirate obtained)	± Fluconazole 400 IV q24 or caspofungin 50 mg IV q24 (guided by culture results)

(Continued)

(Continued)

Site of infection		
Predominant pathogens	Diagnostic investigations	Initial empirical treatment in adult patients

URINARY TRACT INFECTION

Gram-negative bacilli (*Escherichia coli, Klebsiella, Proteus, Enterobacter, Pseudomonas aeruginosa*), *Enterococcus*, coagulase-negative staphylococci, *Candida* spp.	Image kidneys if suspect upper tract infection or graft pyelonephritis. For recurrent UTI, post-void residual urine assessment, cystoscopy, repeat imaging; consider stent removal Remove urinary catheter as soon as non-essential **Note:** If *Staphylococcus aureus* is found in urine culture, the patient should be evaluated for bacteremia	Outpatient therapy: ciprofloxacin 500 mg PO BID *or* amoxicillin/clavulanate 875 mg PO BID *or* cefixime 400 mg PO daily In-patient therapy: piperacillin/tazobactam 3.375 g IV q6h *or* ciprofloxacin 400 mg IV q12h + vancomycin 15 mg/kg IV q12h For *Candida* UTI: fluconazole 200–400 mg PO/IV daily. If azole-resistant, ABLC or L-AmB at 3 mg/kg IV daily or caspofungin 70 mg IV × 1 dose, then 50 mg IV daily (poor urine levels but small case series suggest efficacy). Voriconazole has poor urine levels. Amphotericin bladder washes may be used, although efficacy is unclear.

SKIN AND SOFT TISSUE
Skin and soft tissue infection: Surgical wound infection

Staphylococcus aureus (including MRSA), *Enterococcus* spp., Gram-negative bacilli (Enterobacteriaceae, *Pseudomonas aeruginosa*,) *Candida* spp. Molds, including *Aspergillus* and zygomycetes (uncommon)	Aspiration (needle) or swab of skin exudates for culture Consider imaging to identify deeper abscess	For mild/superficial cellulitis, amoxicillin-clavulanate 875 mg PO BID *or* Cephalexin 500 mg PO QID Consider addition of TMP/SMX double-strength PO BID for MRSA If moderately severe, Vancomycin 15 mg/kg IV q12h ± piperacillin-tazobactam 3.375 g IV q6h

Skin and soft tissue infection: Cellulitis

Staphylococcus aureus, Streptococcus pyogenes, occasionally Gram-negative pathogens Causes of persistent cellulitis include *Cryptococcus*, mycobacteria, molds (e.g. *Aspergillus* and zygomycetes)	If progressive despite empiric treatment, consider imaging and skin biopsy (histology and culture, including fungal, nocardia, AFB); consider serum cryptococcal antigen	Cefazolin 1–2 g IV q8h *or* vancomycin 15 mg/kg IV q12h If diabetic foot ulcer infection, cover for polymicrobial infection (e.g. piperacillin-tazobactam ± vancomycin)

(Continued)

Site of infection		
Predominant pathogens	Diagnostic investigations	Initial empirical treatment in adult patients
Skin and soft tissue infection: papules, nodules		
Disseminated infections: *Candida* spp., *Fusarium* spp., *Cryptococcus*, *Aspergillus*, histoplasmosis, Gram-negative bacilli (*Escherichia coli*, *Pseudomonas aeruginosa*, *Aeromonas hydrophilia*, *Serratia marcescens*), *Nocardia*, atypical mycobacterium, human papillomavirus	Skin biopsy (histopathology; in addition, fresh tissues for aerobic, anaerobic, fungal, *Nocardia*, and AFB cultures) Consider blood cultures × 2, fungal blood culture × 1 if suspect disseminated infection Consider serum cryptococcal antigen, serum galactomannan assay urine histoplasmosis, blastomycosis antigen	Depends on etiology
Skin and soft tissue infection: ulcers, vesicles, hemorrhagic or crusted lesions		
Herpes simplex, VZV, *Staphylococcus aureus*, streptococci	Viral culture, HSV/VZV DFA, or PCR of swab from base of unroofed vesicles	HSV: Valacyclovir 1 g PO BID *or* famciclovir 500 mg PO BID VZV: dermatomal zoster, valacyclovir 1 g PO TID *or* famciclovir 500 PO TID VZV disseminated disease: acyclovir 10 mg/kg IV q8h
Skin and soft tissue infection: skin necrosis		
Aspergillus, Zygomycetes. Embolic phenomenon of endovascular infections of bacterial or fungal etiology, necrotizing fascitis. Pseudomonas, Meningococcus. Other causes of shock, DIC	Blood cultures × 2, including fungal blood culture × 1. Consider serum galactomannan Consider skin biopsy (histology and culture, fungal culture)	Depends on etiology

ABLC, amphotericin B lipid complex; AFB, acid-fast bacilli; ATG, anti-thymocyte globulin; BAL, bronchoalveolar lavage; BID, twice daily; CMV, cytomegalovirus; CNS, central nervous system; CSF, cerebrospinal fluid; CT, computed tomography; CXR, chest X-ray; DFA, direct fluorescent antibody; EBV, Epstein–Barr virus; EIA, enzyme immunoassay; ELISA, enzyme-linked immunosorbent assay; FT-ABS, fluorescent treponemal antibody absorption test; HHV, human herpesvirus; HIV, human immunodeficiency virus; HSV, herpes simplex virus; IgG, immunoglobulin G; IgM, immunoglobulin M; IV, intravenous; L-AmB, liposomal amphotericin B; LCMV, lymphocytic choriomeningitis virus; MAC, *Mycobacterium avium* complex; MMF, mycophenolate mofetil; MRCP, magnetic resonance cholangiopancreatography; MRI, magnetic resonance imaging; NP, nasopharyngeal; O&P, ova and parasite; OPO, organ procurement organization; PCP, *Pneumocystis jirovecii* pneumonia; PO, by mouth; PRES, posterior reversible encephalopathy syndrome; PTLD, post-transplant lymphoproliferative disorder; QID, four times daily; RPR, rapid plasma reagin; SMX, sulfamethoxazole; TB, tuberculosis; TID, three times daily; TMP, trimethoprim; TPN, total parenteral nutrition; UTI, urinary tract infection; VDRL, Venereal Disease Research Laboratory test; VRE, vancomycin-resistant enterococci; VZV, varicella zoster virus; WNV, West Nile virus.

Primary Reference: Glauser MP, Pizzo PA. Management of Infections in Immunocompromised Patients. London: W.B. Saunders Company Ltd, 2000.

8 Management of Infections in Kidney Transplant Recipients[a]

Bartholomew Bono

Syndrome	Microbiology	Therapy	Alternate therapy	Comment
Wound infection	*Staphylococcus aureus*, *Streptococcus* spp.	Vancomycin *or* cefazolin	Clindamycin *or* TMP-SMX	Gram stain and culture of purulent discharge; add anti-GNR therapy if suggested by Gram stain May need to open and debride wound
Infected urinoma or lymphocele	Enterobacteriaceae, enterococci, occasionally yeast	Pip/tazo *or* carbapenem	(Ceftriaxone *or* ceftazidime) + (ampicillin *or* vancomycin)	Drainage with culture and adjust therapy based on results FQ if β-lactam allergy
UTI, including pyelonephritis of allograft – outpatient	Enterobacteriaceae, enterococci, coagulase-negative staphylococci	Oral cephalosporin (second generation: cefuroxime axetil, cefpodoxime) *or* amoxicillin-clavulanate × 2 weeks for graft pyelonephritis	FQ (if not known to harbor FQ-resistant GNRs)	Also do urinalysis FQ resistance on the rise among enteric GNR (center-dependent) TMP-SMX resistance common among SOT recipients because of PCP prophylaxis Perform allograft U/S
UTI, including pyelonephritis of allograft – in-patient	Enterobacteriaceae, enterococci, coagulase-negative staphylococci	Ceftriaxone *or* ceftazidime *or* cefepime *or* pip/tazo *or* carbapenem × 2–3 weeks	If severe sepsis/septic shock, and history of resistant GNRs, empiric carbapenem until culture results known	Also do urinalysis, graft U/S Add ampicillin or vancomycin to treat *Enterococcus* if cephalosporin used FQ resistance on the rise among enteric GNRs (center-dependent) TMP/SMX resistance common among SOT recipients

(Continued)

The AST Handbook of Transplant Infections, 1st edition. Edited by D. Kumar & A. Humar. © 2011 Blackwell Publishing Ltd.

Syndrome	Microbiology	Therapy	Alternate therapy	Comment
Fungal UTI	*Candida* spp. (always treat if symptomatic; many experts will treat even if no symptoms)	Fluconazole × 2–3 weeks	Lipid amphotericin B *or* echinocandin (poor urinary penetration, see comment)	Species identification of yeast is important. Remove urinary catheter. Careful attention to drug-drug interactions if azoles used.[b] Voriconazole poor urine levels Amphotericin bladder washes may be used, although efficacy is unclear
Asymptomatic bacteriuria	Enterobacteriaceae, Enterococci, Coagulase-negative Staphylococci	Observation	Treat based on culture	Some consider treatment of asymptomatic bacteriuria, especially during first 3–6 months post-transplantation
Recurrent UTI	Enterobacteriaceae, enterococci, coagulase-negative staphylococci	Based on cultures; prolonged treatment may be indicated	Prevention: based on cultures, e.g. nitrofurantoin, TMP-SMX, FQ	U/S of graft, removal of ureteral stent if possible. Review hygienic practices; evaluate native kidneys/ ureters; evaluate bladder/ urethra/prostate
Culture-negative graft pyelonephritis	Variable etiologies: fungal, mycobacterial, viral (hemorrhagic; adenovirus, HSV), ureaplasma, *Mycoplasma*	Directed towards pathogen	–	Do fungal, AFB cultures, viral PCR and cultures. Biopsy may be needed
Ureteral ulceration, ureteral stenosis	BK virus (see BK section, Chapter 19)	Reduce immunosuppression	Leflunomide, cidofovir	Tissue needed for definitive diagnosis (urine cytology/ PCR may help)
Nephropathy	BK virus (see BK section, Chapter 19)	Reduce immunosuppression	Leflunomide, cidofovir	Tissue needed for definitive diagnosis (urine cytology/ PCR may help)
Hemorrhagic cystitis	Adenovirus, HSV, BK	Based on etiology	–	BK virus causes hemorrhagic cystitis in HSCT patients but this is rare in SOT Viral urine culture (shell vial); biopsy; PCR on urine, blood or tissue

AFB, acid-fast bacillus; FQ, fluoroquinolone; GNR, gram negative rod; HSCT, hematopoietic stem cell transplant; HSV, herpes simplex virus; PCP, *Pneumocystis carinii* pneumonia; PCR, polymerase chain reaction; pip/tazo, piperacillin-tazobactam. SOT, solid organ transplant; TMP-SMX, trimethoprim-sulfamethoxazole; U/S, ultrasound; UTI, urinary tract infection
[a]Management suggestions assume a high prevalence of methicillin-resistant *Staphylococcus aureus* (MRSA), FQ- and TMP-SMX-resistant GNRs.
[b]Caspofungin 70 mg IV x 1 dose, then 50 mg IV daily (poor urine levels but small case series).

9 Management of Infections in Pancreas Transplant Recipients [a, b] [1–3]

Bartholomew Bono

Syndrome	Microbiology	Therapy	Alternate therapy	Comment
Wound infection	*Staphylococcus aureus*, *Streptococcus* spp.	Vancomycin *or* cefazolin	Clindamycin *or* TMP-SMX	Gram stain and culture of purulent discharge; add anti-GNR therapy if suggested by Gram stain May need to open and debride wound
Pancreatic abscess	Enterobacteriaceae, enterococci, anaerobes, *Candida* spp.	Pip/tazo *or* (ceftazidime + metronidazole) *or* (cefepime + metronidazole) *and* fluconazole	(Carbapenem *or* tigecycline) + (fluconazole *or* echinocandin)	Percutaneous drainage ± surgical debridement High rate of *Candida* infection Add vancomycin if Gram-positive cocci on Gram stain Assess vasculature
Peritonitis or intra-abdominal abscess	Enterobacteriaceae, enterococci, anaerobes, *Candida* spp.	Pip/tazo *or* (ceftazidime + metronidazole) *or* (cefepime + metronidazole) *and* fluconazole	(Carbapenem *or* tigecycline[c]) + (fluconazole *or* echinocandin)	Rule out anastomotic leaks/ bowel perforation (see section 6.1)

GNR, gram negative rod; pip/tazo, piperacillin-tazobactam; TMP-SMX, trimethoprim- sulfamethoxazole.
[a]Management suggestions assume a high prevalence of methicillin-resistant *Staphylococcus aureus* (MRSA), fluoroquinolone- and TMP/SMX-resistant GNRs.
[b]Recipients of simultaneous kidney–pancreas transplants generally have higher infection rates than kidney alone.
[c]There has been an FDA warning in 2010 about potential for increased mortality with tigecycline in severe infections.

References (in square brackets): [1] *Nephrol Dial Transplant* 1997; 12(4): 764: [2] *Am J Surg* 2000; 179(2): 99; [3] *Ann Surg* 2001; 233(4): 463.

The AST Handbook of Transplant Infections, 1st edition. Edited by D. Kumar & A. Humar. © 2011 Blackwell Publishing Ltd.

10 Management of Infections in Liver Transplant Recipients [a] [1–3]

Bartholomew Bono

Syndrome	Microbiology	Therapy	Alternate therapy	Comment
Wound infection	*Staphylococcus aureus*, *Streptococcus* spp., less likely Enterobacteriaceae, anaerobes	Vancomycin or cefazolin	If drug resistance or Gram-negative organisms suspected: (pip/tazo or carbapenem) ± vancomycin	Gram stain and culture of purulent discharge. Note preoperative colonization with MRSA, VRE, resistant GNRs May need to open and debride wound
Infected biloma/bile leak/secondary peritonitis	Enterococci, Enterobacteriaceae, coagulase-negative staphylococci, *Candida* spp.	Vancomycin + (pip/tazo or carbapenem) + fluconazole	Substitute linezolid for vancomycin if high rate of VRE Echinocandin is an alternative to fluconazole	Percutaneous and/or surgical drainage and correction of leak Tigecycline is an option for those with β-lactam allergy[b] Secondary prophylaxis usually associated with bile leak, bowel perforation or other technical problems
Cholangitis	Enterobacteriaceae, enterococci, anaerobes, *Candida* spp.	(Vancomycin + pip/tazo or carbapenem) or (vancomycin + ceftriaxone + metronidazole)	Vancomycin + (FQ or aztreonam) + metronidazole	Assess adequacy of biliary tree/check for strictures (U/S, CT, PTC and/or MRCP) Tigecycline is an option for those with β-lactam allergy[b] Add antifungal if there is high suspicion for fungal infection
Hepatic abscess	Enterobacteriaceae, enterococci, anaerobes, *Candida* spp.	(Vancomycin + pip/tazo or carbapenem) or (vancomycin + ceftriaxone + metronidazole)	Vancomycin + (FQ or aztreonam) + metronidazole	Percutaneous drainage Rule out hepatic artery thrombosis Add antifungal if *Candida* spp. Is suggested by Gram stain Amebic liver abscess rare after liver transplantation
Fever early post-liver transplant (< 3 weeks)	Depends on source (see comment)	Empiric antimicrobial therapy usually indicated	–	Evaluation includes abdominal imaging (U/S and/or CT scan), including graft, hepatic artery assessment. Rule out biloma

(Continued)

The AST Handbook of Transplant Infections, 1st edition. Edited by D. Kumar & A. Humar. © 2011 Blackwell Publishing Ltd.

(*Continued*)

Syndrome	Microbiology	Therapy	Alternate therapy	Comment
Hepatic artery thrombosis (HAT)	As above	Thrombectomy if detected early	Re-transplantation may be required	May range from asymptomatic to severe hepatic necrosis Common complications include biliary leak, strictures, hepatic abscess. Treat complications with antimicrobials as above
Hepatitis	CMV, HBV, HCV	Treatment depends on pathogen, see specific sections	–	–
Hepatitis	Adenovirus	Cidofovir	Ganciclovir (may be active against some serotypes)	Reduce immunosuppression

CMV, cytomegalovirus; CT, computed tomography; FQ, fluoroquinolone; GNR, gram negative rod; HBV, hepatitis B virus; HCV, hepatitis C virus; MRCP, magnetic resonance cholangiopancreatography; MRSA, methicillin-resistant *Staphylococcus aureus*; pip/tazo, piperacillin-tazobactam; PTC, percutaneous transhepatic cholangiogram; U/S, ultrasound; VRE, vancomycin-resistant enterococci.

[a]Management suggestions assume a high prevalence of MRSA, FQ- and trimethoprim-sulfamethoxazole (TMP/SMX)-resistant GNRs.

[b]There has been an FDA warning in 2010 about potential for increased mortality with tigecycline in severe infections.

References: [1] *Liver Transpl* 2006; 12(8): 1244; [2] *Clin Infect Dis* 2004;39(4):517; [3] *Transplantation* 2003; 75(1): 79.

11 Management of Infections in Lung, Heart–Lung, and Heart Transplant Recipients

Shahid Husain & S.M. Hosseini-Mogaddham

Syndrome	Etiology	Preferred regimen	Alternative regimen	Comments
Lung transplant perioperative prophylaxis	Based on pre-transplant colonization and donor respiratory colonization	Non-CF: second- or third-generation cephalosporin or pip/tazo × 48–72 h CF, *cepacia*-negative: based on pre-transplant culture results CF, *cepacia*-positive: based on pre-transplant MCBT	Non-CF: levofloxacin + vancomycin CF, *cepacia*-negative: ceftazidime + meropenem + inhaled tobramycin CF, *cepacia*-positive: meropenem + ceftazidime + inhaled tobramycin + levofloxacin	Adjust antibiotics based on donor respiratory culture results.
Bacterial pneumonia or bacterial tracheobronchitis	*Staphylococcus aureus*, Enterobacteriaceae, *Pseudomonas aeruginosa*, other Gram-negatives, *B. cepacia* (in *cepacia*+ CF lung transplants)	Vancomycin 1 g q12h + pip/tazo 4.5 g, q8h + azithromycin 500 mg/day × 14–21 days	Linezolid 600 mg BID + ciprofloxacin 400 mg IV q8h or levofloxacin 750 mg IV	In lung transplant, rule out non-infectious causes (rejection, reperfusion injury) Combination therapy for suspected Gram-negative infection during early transplant (< 1 month) is recommended empirically (β-lactam + aminoglycoside ± fluoroquinolone) based on susceptibility. Combination therapy for Gram- positives not recommended
Burkholderia cepacia infection in CF lung transplant –pneumonia, empyema, bacteremia, metastatic abscess, wound infection	*B. cepacia* complex	Tobramycin 4–7 mg/kg/dose once daily + meropenem 1 g q8h + ceftazidime 2 g q8h	Two- to four-drug regimen based on sensitivities and MCBT testing (see comment). Other potential antibiotics include: cefepime, TMP-SMX, FQ, colistin, azithromycin, other aminoglycosides, pip/tazo, aztreonam	MCBT or synergy testing is routinely employed to design treatment combinations for CF patients Recipients infected with Bcc, subspecies *B. cenocepacia* have considerably worse graft survival Adjunctive surgical therapy may be required

(Continued)

The AST Handbook of Transplant Infections, 1st edition. Edited by D. Kumar & A. Humar. © 2011 Blackwell Publishing Ltd.

(*Continued*)

Syndrome	Etiology	Preferred regimen	Alternative regimen	Comments
Bacterial colonization Presence of positive BAL bacterial culture without clinical or radiological findings	Prevalence is around 40% Mostly Gram-negatives followed by Gram-positive organism	Similar to bacterial pneumonia	Similar to bacterial pneumonia	Bacterial colonization is associated with lower O$_2$ index in the first 6 hours, longer ICU stay, prolonged mechanical ventilation, and lower graft survival The risk of progression to pneumonia is high in lung transplant
Fungal colonization, lung transplant – Candida	Most prevalent species is *C. albicans* followed by *C. glabrata*, *C. parapsilosis* and *C. tropicalis*	Fluconazole 400 mg once daily (treat only if recent lung transplant and persistent heavy growth).	Inhaled amphotericin B 10 mg bid (± bronchodilator)	Do not recommend prophylaxis once the bronchial anastomosis has healed Use of anti-*Aspergillus* prophylaxis will also cover
Fungal colonization, lung transplant – mold	Most common species *A. fumigatus* followed by *A. niger*, *A. flavus* and *A. terreus* Non-*Aspergillus* molds Incidence up to 14%	Inhaled amphotericin B 20 mg BID (± bronchodilator) *or* Voriconazole 200 mg PO BID	Inhaled ABLC 50 mg/day × 4 days followed by 50 mg/week for at least 7 weeks Inhaled L-AmB 25 mg three times/week for the first 60 days after transplantation, 25 mg/week between 60 and 180 days, and 25 mg once every 2 weeks thereafter Itraconazole 200 mg PO BID	Recommended during the first year after lung transplantation. Patients with pre-transplant *Aspergillus* colonization are also recommended to receive prophylaxis Inhaled L-AmB had lower side-effect profile than inhaled amphotericin B deoxycholate Use of azoles requires hepatic enzyme monitoring and adjustment of the dose of calcineurin inhibitors by 50% For non-*Aspergillus* mold colonization, may need alternative therapy based on species
Fungal pneumonia and tracheobronchitis	*A. fumigatus* followed by *A. niger*, *A. flavus* and *A. terreus*. The majority of *Aspergillus* infection tends to occur after 1 year of transplant	Voriconazole (6 mg/kg IV q12h × 1 day, then 4 mg/kg IV q12h) *or* Oral loading 300–400 mg PO BID × 1 day, then 200 mg PO BID × 12 weeks minimum	L-AmB (3–5 mg/kg/day IV) *or* ABLC (5 mg/kg/day IV) *or* caspofungin (70 mg IV on day 1, then 50 mg/day IV) *or* micafungin (IV 100–150 mg/day) *or* posaconazole (200 mg QID initially, then 400 mg BID PO after stabilization of disease)	BAL galactomannan is more sensitive than serum galactomannan

Syndrome	Etiology	Preferred regimen	Alternative regimen	Comments
	Lung transplants have risk of other molds including *Zygomycetes*, *Scedosporium* and others (see Chapter 25)	Consider combination therapy with echinocandin for more severe disease Consider inhaled amphotericin products for adjunctive therapy of tracheobronchitis		Bronchoscopic debridement for necrotic debris at the site of bronchial anastomosis Consider reducing immunosuppression Consider combination therapy in patients who develop invasive aspergillosis early during transplantation and are in ICU Consider therapeutic drug monitoring for voriconazole if available
Toxoplasmosis in heart/heart–lung transplant patients – includes disseminated disease, CNS disease, pneumonitis	*Toxoplasma gondii* Prophylaxis (D+/R−): TMP-SMX one tablet DS[a] daily or three times/week *or* Pyrimethamine alone	Pyrimethamine (200 mg loading dose PO then 75 mg/day) + sulfadiazine (1–1.5 g PO q6h) + folinic acid PO 10–25 mg/day	Pyrimethamine (200 mg loading dose PO then 75 mg/day) + clindamycin (600 mg IV or 450 mg PO q6h) + folinic acid PO 10–25 mg/day *or* Atovaquone (1500 mg PO BID)	Transmission rate is high in mismatched D+/R− heart or heart-lung transplant recipients, low in R+ Recommend donor and recipient screening at the time of transplant for heart
Empyema	*S. aureus*, *Pseudomonas*, *Candida*. If *cepacia* + CF, then empyema is usually due to *B. cepacia*. Other rare causes include *Mycoplasma*, *Nocardia*, *Cryptococcus*, *Legionella*, *Aspergillus*, *Mycobacteria*	Pip/tazo + vancomycin + fluconazole (if possibility of aspergillosis then voriconazole)	Vancomycin + carbapenem + fluconazole	Chest tube drainage Intrapleural fibrinolysis is not recommended Video-assisted thoracoscopic surgery (VATS) in cases with loculated empyema Early onset (<14 days after lung surgeries) is commonly associated with a bronchopleural fistula Antibiotic irrigation, surgical closure of bronchopleural fistulae

(Continued)

(Continued)

Syndrome	Etiology	Preferred regimen	Alternative regimen	Comments
Mediastinitis	*S. aureus*, coagulase-negative *Staphylococcus*, *Enterobacter*, *Acinetobacter*, *Klebsiella*, *Aspergillus* If *cepacia* + CF, then mediastinitis is usually due to *B. cepacia*	Vancomycin + pip/tazo × 4–6 weeks	Vancomycin + carbapenem	CT-guided percutaneous drainage Switch to specific regimen based on cultures Sternal and mediastinal debridement with rewiring of the sternum
CMV pneumonitis	CMV	Ganciclovir 5 mg/kg IV q12 h	Valganciclovir 900 mg PO BID (usually only for mild pneumonitis or step-down after clinical improvement)	See specific details in CMV section (Chapter 14) Lung transplant patients are at high risk of CMV and have higher risk of ganciclovir resistance (see Chapter 14) Consider CMV Ig especially in D+/R−
Respiratory viruses	Influenza, RSV, parainfluenza, adenovirus, human metapneumovirus, rhinovirus, coronavirus	Treatment based on specific pathogen (see Chapter 20)	Corticosteroids are sometimes used as adjunctive therapy in lung transplant patients	Respiratory viruses are implicated in the development of bronchiolitis obliterans syndrome (lung transplant). Many experts treat aggressively despite lack of evidence or proven antivirals for many pathogens
Nocardia	See specific table for *Nocardia* (Chapter 26)			3.5% in lung transplants and 2.5% in heart transplants

ABLC, amphotericin B lipid complex; BAL, bronchoalveolar lavage; Bcc, burkholderia cepacia complex; BID, twice daily; CF, cystic fibrosis; CMV, cytomegalovirus; CNS, central nervous system; CT, computed tomography; D+/R−, donor positive/recipient negative; FQ, fluoroquinolone; Ig, immunoglobulin; IV, intravenous; L-AmB, liposomal amphotericin B; MCBT, multiple combination bactericidal antibiotic testing; pip/tazo, piperacillin-tazobactam; PO, by mouth; R+, recipient positive; RSV, respiratory syncytial virus; TMP-SMX, trimethoprim- sulfamethoxazole.

[a]DS, double strength: TMP, 160 mg/SMX, 800 mg.

12 Management of Infections in Intestinal Transplant Recipients[a]

Michael Green

Syndrome	Microbiology	Suggested empiric therapy	Alternate therapy	Comment
Surgical site infection	*Staphylococcus aureus*, *Streptococcus* spp., less likely Enterobacteriaceae, anaerobes	Vancomycin + (pip/taz *or* cefepime *or* carbapenem)	clindamycin ± (AG *or* aztreonam)	Gram stain and culture of purulent discharge. Note preoperative colonization with MRSA, VRE, resistant GNRs. Use of cefepime is preferred over ceftazidime secondary to high prevalence of ampC β-lactamase producing GNR
Intra-abdominal abscess	Enterobacteriaceae, enterococci, anaerobes, *Candida* spp.	Pip/taz *or* Cefepime *or* carbapenem ± antifungal (see comment)	Quinolone *or* tigecycline[b] Use of AG is limited secondary to potential toxicity	Add fluconazole or echinocandin if *Candida* spp. is suggested by Gram stain or consider adding empirically; add vancomycin if GPC is morphologically consistent with *Staphylococcus*. Consider use of linezolid if there is a history of VRE colonization. Use of cefepime is preferred over ceftazidime secondary to high prevalence of ampC β-lactamase producing GNR
Peritonitis, secondary	Enterobacteriaceae, enterococci, anaerobes, *Candida* spp.	Pip/taz *or* Cefepime *or* carbapenem ± antifungal (see comment)	Quinolone *or* tigecycline[b] Use of AG is limited secondary to potential toxicity	Gram stain and culture of purulent material. Usually associated with biliary leak, intra-abdominal bleeding, biliary stricture, or bowel leak or perforation Same comments as for intra-abdominal abscess
Bloodstream infection – gut-associated	Enterobacteriaceae, enterococci; less likely yeast	Vancomycin + (pip/taz *or* cefepime *or* carbapenem)	Quinolone *or* tigecycline[b] Use of AG is limited secondary to potential toxicity	Typically seen in patients with underlying disease of intestinal mucosa (e.g. PTLD, rejection, GVHD). Can be seen early or late post-transplant dependent upon status of intestinal mucosa. Empiric therapy should take into consideration prior history of colonization with VRE, resistant GNR
Urinary tract infection	Enterobacteriaceae, enterococci; less likely yeast	Pip/taz *or* cefepime	TMP-SMX if active; quinolone or carbapenem	–

(Continued)

The AST Handbook of Transplant Infections, 1st edition. Edited by D. Kumar & A. Humar. © 2011 Blackwell Publishing Ltd.

(*Continued*)

Syndrome	Microbiology	Suggested empiric therapy	Alternate therapy	Comment
Enteritis	*Clostridium difficile*	PO metronidazole *or* PO vancomycin	PO vancomycin may be preferred for severe disease. Use of IV metronidazole may be added in this scenario	Consideration of combination therapy for severe or life-threatening disease. May require prolonged therapy for those with recurrent disease
Enteritis	CMV	IV ganciclovir	CMV-IV Ig may be used in addition to ganciclovir	CMV enteritis is the most common site of tissue-invasive CMV disease in intestinal transplant. May see histologic evidence of disease in the absence of measurable CMV load in the peripheral blood
Enteritis/PTLD	EBV	Reduce immunosuppression	IV ganciclovir ± IV Ig is often used but is of unproven benefit Rituximab may be used especially if reduction of immunosuppression is not possible (e.g. concurrent rejection)	EBV in intestinal transplant recipients is frequently limited to intestinal involvement only. Frequent presence of EBV-infected B cells in intestines (native and allograft) in the absence of proven disease. EBV load measured by NAT of blood may be useful for both diagnosis and assessment of clinical response
Enteritis	Adenovirus	Cidofovir	–	Need to differentiate between symptomatic enteritis and localized reactivation, which is often asymptomatic and self-limited. Measurement of adenovirus load in the blood by NAT may be of value for diagnosis of disease and for following patient

AG, aminoglycosides; ampC, CMV, cytomegalovirus; EBV, Epstein–Barr virus; GNR, Gram Negative Rods; GPC, Gram-positive cocci; GVHD, graft-versus-host disease; MRSA, methicillin-resistant *Staphylococcus aureus*; NAT, nucleic acid testing; pip/tazo, piperacillin-tazobactam; PTLD, post-transplant lymphoproliferative disorder; TMP-SMX, trimethoprim-sulfamethoxazole; VRE, vancomycin-resistant enterococci.

[a]Suggested therapies are based on a high prevalence of MRSA, VRE, multi-drug-resistant GNRs. Local prevalence may vary.
[b]There has been an FDA warning in 2010 about potential for increased mortality with tigecycline in severe infections.

References: [1] *Am J Transplantation* 2007; 7(5 Pt 2): 1376; [2] *Am J Transplantation* 2005; 5: 1430; [3] *Ann Surgery* 2006; 243: 756; [4] *Transplantation* 2000; 70(2): 302; [5] *Curr Opin Organ Transpl* 1999; 4: 361.

13 Antimicrobial Management of Patients with Fever and Neutropenia Following Hematopoietic Stem Cell Transplantation

Upton D. Allen

13.1 Stepwise approach to empiric antimicrobial therapy in febrile neutropenia[a]

Step	Therapy	Notes
Step 1: Initial therapy	Anti-pseudomonal beta-lactam (e.g. piperacillin-tazobactam) + aminoglycoside	Alternatives: monotherapy - piperacillin-tazobactam, cefepime or a carbapenem. Other agents may be used as part of the initial regimen (e.g., fluoroquinolones or vancomycin) depending on the presence of complications (e.g., hypotension) or if there are specific concerns about antimicrobial resistance.
Step 2: Afebrile within first 3 days	*No etiology identified:* Low risk[c] – change to an oral agent (e.g. amoxicillin-clavulanate + ciprofloxacin) High risk – continue same antibiotics *Etiology identified:* adjust to most appropriate treatment	
Step 3: Persistent fever during first 3–5 days	*If no clinical change:* continue antibiotics; consider stopping vancomycin if cultures are negative	
	If progressive disease: change antibiotics and add antifungal therapy (see Section 13.2)	Regimens vary and depend on local flora. Broader and/or a different class of antibiotics may be used
Step 4: Persistent fever after 5–7 days	Consider adding antifungal therapy ± antibiotic changes	Fungal work-up initiated at days 4-5 (e.g. CT chest/abdomen, serum galactomannan). Some experts will start antifungal therapy earlier, e.g. at day 3 For antifungal agents, see Section 13.2
Step 5: Reassess duration of antimicrobial therapy	Duration of antimicrobials is dependent on neutrophil recovery and whether etiology was identified	Antibiotics should be continued for at least the duration of neutropenia. Longer durations may be required as clinically indicated.

ANC, Absolute neutrophil count; CT, computed tomography.

[a]Fever is defined as single oral temperature of ≥ 38.3 °C or a temperature of ≥ 38.0 °C for at least 1 hour. Neutropenia is defined as a count < 0.5 × 10^9/L add cells/L. The units should be × 10^9 cells/L or an ANC that is expected to decrease to < 0.5 × 10^9/L during the next 48 hours.

[b]Vancomycin use is indicated if there is severe mucositis, obvious catheter-related infection, hypotension, prior colonization with MRSA or penicillin/cephalosporin-resistant pneumococci, recent or current fluoroquinolone prophylaxis.

[c]Indicators of high-risk for severe infection include: anticipated prolonged (>7 days duration) and profound neutropenia (ANC < 0.1 × 10^9 cells/L) and/or co-morbid conditions, including hypotension, pneumonia, new-onset abdominal pain, or neurologic changes.

The AST Handbook of Transplant Infections, 1st edition. Edited by D. Kumar & A. Humar. © 2011 Blackwell Publishing Ltd.

13.2 **Agents for empiric antifungal therapy in febrile neutropenia**

Acceptable agents	Comments

Lipid amphotericn B products
   Amphotericin B lipid complex
   Liposomal amphotericin B
	Conventional amphotericin B is usually not preferred post-HSCT due to nephrotoxicity and less evidence of efficacy

Echinocandins
   Caspofungin
   Micafungin
	The echinocandins are favored in patients with renal impairment or are intolerant of amphotericin products

Azoles
   Voriconazole
   Posaconazole
	Fluconazole is often used as prophylaxis HSCT patients. This limits its used for empiric therapy in persistently febrile neutropenics

	More pediatric data are required for posaconazole

HSCT, hematopoietic stem cell transplant.
Freifeld AG, et al. Clinical Practice Guideline for the use of Antimicrobial Agents in Neutropenic Patients with Cancer: 2010 update by the Infectious Diseases Society of America. CID 2011;52(4):e56–e93.

PART II
Specific Pathogens

14 Cytomegalovirus

Raymund R. Razonable & Atul Humar

14.1 Prevention of cytomegalovirus (CMV) disease in solid organ transplant (SOT) recipients

Type of transplant/modi-fying circumstance	Primary (preferred) strategy and agent(s)[a]	Alternative strategy and agent(s)	Comments
Kidney, liver, pancreas, and heart			
D+/R−	Antiviral prophylaxis is preferred: valganciclovir, 900 mg PO daily × 3–6 months	Antiviral prophylaxis: ganciclovir 1 g PO TID, valacyclovir 2 g PO QID (for kidney recipients only)	Valganciclovir is not FDA-approved for liver transplant recipients, but it is still the most commonly used drug for prophylaxis
		Pre-emptive therapy: val-ganciclovir 900 mg PO BID or ganciclovir 5 mg/kg IV BID for positive CMV PCR or antigen-emia test (see pre-emptive algorithm, Fig. 14.3)	Late-onset CMV disease is the major complication of prophylaxis; occurring in 10–36% of D+/R− patients [1]
		Some centers add CMVIg for heart recipients	Six months of valganciclovir prophylaxis had improved efficacy vs 3 months in kidney [2]
			Leukopenia and neutropenia are common with ganciclovir and valganciclovir. Neurologic toxicity occurs with high-dose valacyclovir [3]
R+	Antiviral prophylaxis: valganciclovir, 900 mg PO daily × 3 months	Ganciclovir 1 g PO TID, valacyclovir 2 g PO QID (for kidney recipients only)	Prophylaxis may be preferred if ALG or alemtuzumab is used for induc-tion therapy
	or	*or*	Low risk of late-onset CMV disease compared with D+/R− patients
	Pre-emptive therapy (see pre-emptive algorithm, Fig. 14.3)	Pre-emptive therapy (see pre-emptive algorithm, Fig. 14.3)	Leukopenia and neutropenia are common with ganciclovir and valganciclovir. Neurologic toxicity occurs with high-dose valacyclovir [3]
			Oral ganciclovir and valacyclovir should not be used for pre-emptive therapy

(Continued)

The AST Handbook of Transplant Infections, 1st edition. Edited by D. Kumar & A. Humar. © 2011 Blackwell Publishing Ltd.

(Continued)

Type of transplant/modifying circumstance	Primary (preferred) strategy and agent(s)[a]	Alternative strategy and agent(s)	Comments
Lung (and heart–lung)			
D+/R−	Antiviral prophylaxis is preferred: valganciclovir 900 mg PO daily × 6–12 months	Antiviral prophylaxis: ganciclovir 5 mg/kg IV daily. Some centers add unselected or CMVIg [4]	Oral ganciclovir is not recommended because of poor absorption and the risk of drug resistance development. Many centers start with IV ganciclovir and then transition to valganciclovir. 12 months' prophylaxis was superior to 3 months in a multicenter trial [5]
R+	Antiviral prophylaxis is preferred: valganciclovir, 900 mg PO QD × 3–6 months	Antiviral prophylaxis is preferred: ganciclovir 5 mg/kg IV daily, ganciclovir 1 g PO TID *or* Pre-emptive therapy (see pre-emptive algorithm, Fig. 14.3)	CMV R+ lung transplant recipients are considered as high risk, and antiviral prophylaxis is preferred. Oral ganciclovir is generally not preferred because of poor absorption and the risk of drug resistance development. Some centers will prolong prophylaxis to 12 months [5]
Intestinal			
D+/R− or R+	Antiviral prophylaxis is preferred: ganciclovir 5 mg/kg IV daily × 3–6 months	Ganciclovir 5 mg/kg IV daily, then switch to valganciclovir 900 mg PO daily × 3–6 months total if graft function is adequate. Some centers add unselected or CMVIg for D+/R−	Pharmacokinetics of oral valganciclovir are not defined in intestinal recipients. CMV R+ intestinal transplant recipients are considered as high risk, and antiviral prophylaxis is preferred
All organs			
Treatment of acute rejection (especially if ALG used)	Antiviral prophylaxis is preferred: valganciclovir 900 mg PO daily	Antiviral prophylaxis: ganciclovir 5 mg/kg IV daily. Preiemptive therapy (see pre-emptive algorithm, Fig. 14.3)	High risk of CMV reactivation during treatment of acute rejection, especially with lymphocyte-depleting agents in D+/R− patients. Duration of antiviral prophylaxis is 2–4 weeks

(Continued)

Type of transplant/modifying circumstance	Primary (preferred) strategy and agent(s)[a]	Alternative strategy and agent(s)	Comments
Prevention of late-onset CMV disease	Extend prophylaxis (e.g. from 3 months to 6 months)	Close clinical follow-up	Mostly a problem in D+/R− recipients
	or		
	Viral load or antigenemia monitoring after completing prophylaxis (e.g. weekly × 8 weeks)		
D−/R−	Use CMV-negative and/or leukodepleted blood products		Most centers will not use CMV-specific prophylaxis for this subgroup of patients

ALG, anti-lymphocyte globulin; BID, twice daily; CMV, cytomegalovirus; D+/R−, donor positive/recipient negative; Ig, immunoglobulin; IV, intravenous; PO, by mouth; QD, once a day; QID, four times daily; R+, recipient positive; TID, three times daily.

[a]Drug doses provided should be adjusted based on creatinine clearance:

- Ganciclovir IV: *prophylaxis* – creatinine clearance (CrCl – ml/min) > 70: 5 mg/kg q24 h; CrCl 50–69: 2.5 mg/kg q24 h; CrCl 25–49: 1.25 mg/kg q24 h; CrCl 10–24: 0.625 mg/kg q24 h; CrCl < 10 or hemodialysis: 0.625 mg/kg three times weekly; continuous renal replacement therapy (CRRT): 5 mg/kg q24 h; *pre-emptive therapy* – CrCl > 70: 5 mg/kg q12 h; CrCl 50–69: 2.5 mg/kg q12 h; CrCl 25–49: 2.5 mg/kg q24 h; CrCl 10–24: 1.25 mg/kg q24 h; CrCl < 10 or hemodialysis: 1.25 mg/kg three times weekly; CRRT: 2.5 mg/kg q24 h.
- Valganciclovir PO: *prophylaxis* – CrCl > 60: 900 mg PO QD; CrCl 40–59: 450 mg QD; CrCl 25–39: 450 mg q48 h; CrCl 10–24: 450 mg twice weekly; CrCl < 10 and hemodialysis: not recommended; *pre-emptive therapy* – CrCl > 60: 900 mg PO BID; CrCl 40–59: 450 mg BID; CrCl 25–39: 450 mg q24 h; CrCl 10–24: 450 mg q48 h; CrCl < 10 and hemodialysis: not recommended.
- Ganciclovir PO: *prophylaxis* – CrCl > 70: 1 g TID; CrCl 50–69: 500 mg TID; CrCl 25–49: 500 mg BID; CrCl 10–24: 500 mg QD; CrCl < 10 and intermittent hemodialysis: 500 mg three times weekly; *pre-emptive therapy* – not recommended.

Foscarnet and cidofovir are generally not recommended for primary prophylaxis because of high risk of toxicity.

References (in square brackets): [1] *Am J Transplantation* 2009; **9**(s4): S78; [2] *Am J Transplantation* 2010; **10**(5):1228; [3] *New Engl J Med* 1999; **340**(19): 1462; [4] *Transplantation* 2005; **80**(2): 157; [5] *Ann Int Med* 2010: **152**(12): 761.

14.2 Interpretation of pediatric CMV serology in donors and recipients <18 months[a] [1]

	CMV serology positive and culture negative or unavailable	CMV serology negative and culture negative or unavailable	CMV culture positive
Donor <18 months of age: check urine/throat culture if possible	Assumption = *positive* (even though this may be false positive due to maternal transfer)	Assumption = *negative*	Assumption = *positive* (regardless of serology)
Recipient <18 months of age: check urine/throat culture if possible	Assumption = *negative* (if donor is seropositive) Assumption = *positive* (if donor is seronegative)	Assumption = *negative*	Assumption = *positive* (regardless of serology)

[a]Serology at less than 18 months of age may not be reliable due to passive transfer of antibody. The above assumptions are made to assign the highest-risk donor/recipient serostatus to the transplant patient.

Reference (in square brackets): [1] *Transplantation* 2010; **89**(7): 779.

14.3 Algorithm for pre-emptive therapy of CMV in organ transplant recipients

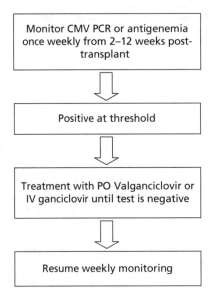

Notes:

1. Pre-emptive is therapy better suited for low-risk patients.
2. Thresholds are assay-dependent and also organ/D/R serostatus/immunosuppression risk-dependent, e.g. a lower threshold may be used for D+/R−, lung transplant recipient, recent induction immunosuppression. Commonly used thresholds for CMV antigenemia assay may be 5–10 per 100 000 cells, and 1000 copies/mL for plasma CMV PCR by Roche Amplicor assay.
3. Recurrent CMV viremia may occur, requiring repeated therapy.

14.4 Treatment of CMV infection and disease in SOT recipients

Type of CMV disease Preferred/first-line agent[a,b]	Alternative drugs[c]	Comments
Asymptomatic CMV infection/viremia[d]		
Valganciclovir 900 mg PO BID	Ganciclovir 5 mg/kg IV q12h	Consider reducing immunosuppression[e]
		Monitor viral load or antigenemia once weekly
		Duration of treatment is individualized, and preferably until 2 weeks after clearance of viremia
CMV syndrome[f]		
Valganciclovir 900 mg PO BID	Foscarnet IV 60 mg/kg q8h or 90 mg/kg q12h	Consider reducing immunosuppression
or	*or*	Duration of treatment is individualized, and preferably until 2 weeks after clearance of viremia and clinical resolution (1–3)
Ganciclovir 5 mg/kg IV q12h	Cidofovir IV 5 mg/kg weekly × 2 weeks and every 2 weeks thereafter	
If starting with IV ganciclovir, may switch to valganciclovir when clinically and virologically improving		

(Continued)

Type of CMV disease Preferred/first-line agent[a,b]	Alternative drugs[c]	Comments
Tissue-invasive CMV disease		
Ganciclovir 5 mg/kg IV q12 h Valganciclovir 900 mg PO BID (do not use oral therapy if there is malabsorption or severe disease) May start with IV ganciclovir and switch to valganciclovir when clinically and virologically improving	Foscarnet 60 mg/kg q8 h or 90 mg/kg q12 h *or* Cidofovir 5 mg/kg weekly × 2 weeks and every 2 weeks thereafter	Reduce immunosuppression Duration of treatment is individualized, and usually prolonged. Treat until 2 weeks after clinical and virologic clearance of infection [1–3] Some cases of tissue-invasive CMV disease are compartmentalized (e.g. enteritis), and CMV testing in the blood may not reflect extent of disease
CMV pneumonia		
Ganciclovir 5 mg/kg IV q12 h	Foscarnet IV 60 mg/kg q8 h or 90 mg/kg q12 h *or* Cidofovir 5 mg/kg weekly for 2 weeks and every 2 weeks thereafter	Reduce immunosuppression Valganciclovir is not preferred as first line because of the potentially severe and fatal outcome of CMV pneumonia. May transition IV ganciclovir to valganciclovir 900 mg PO BID when clinically stable Some add CMVIg (e.g., Cytogam® 100–150 mg/kg three times per week) especially if clinically severe
Gastrointestinal CMV disease		
Ganciclovir 5 mg/kg IV q12 h	Valganciclovir 900 mg PO BID *or* Foscarnet 60 mg/kg q8 h or 90 mg/kg q12 h *or* Cidofovir 5 mg/kg weekly for 2 weeks and every 2 weeks thereafter	Reduce immunosuppression Valganciclovir is not preferred as first-line agent in severe cases of gastrointestinal disease due to concerns with absorption. May transition from IV ganciclovir to valganciclovir 900 mg PO BID when clinically stable Some cases of gastrointestinal CMV disease are compartmentalized, and CMV testing in the blood may not reflect extent of disease
CMV retinitis		
Ganciclovir 5 mg/kg IV q12 h *or* Valganciclovir 900 mg PO BID	Intravitreal ganciclovir or fomivirsen (consult opthalomologist) *and/or* Foscarnet IV 60 mg/kg q8 h or 90 mg/kg q12 h *or* Cidofovir IV 5 mg/kg × 2 weeks and every 2 weeks thereafter	Reduce immunosuppression Duration of treatment is guided by repeat fundoscopic examination by ophthalmologist
CMV CNS disease		
Ganciclovir 5 mg/kg IV q12 h	Foscarnet IV 60 mg/kg q8 h or 90 mg/kg q12 h *or* Cidofovir IV 5 mg/kg weekly for 2 weeks and every 2 weeks thereafter	Reduce immunosuppression IV ganciclovir is recommended over valganciclovir as first line so that immediate high systemic levels are achieved

(Continued)

(*Continued*)

Type of CMV disease Preferred/first-line agent[a,b]	Alternative drugs[c]	Comments
Severe CMV disease[g]		
Ganciclovir 5 mg/kg IV q12 h	Foscarnet IV 60 mg/kg q8 h or 90 mg/kg q12 h	Reduce immunosuppression
	or	Some add CMVIg (e.g. Cytogam 100–150 mg/kg three times per week)
	Cidofovir IV 5 mg/kg weekly × 2 weeks and every 2 weeks thereafter	Valganciclovir has not been studied for treatment of severe CMV disease
		May transition from IV ganciclovir to valganciclovir 900 mg PO BID when clinically stable
Ganciclovir-resistant CMV disease (see Fig. 14.5)		
Reduce immunosuppression	Cidofovir 5 mg/kg weekly × 2 weeks and every 2 weeks thereafter	Test for *UL97* and *UL54* gene mutation to guide treatment choice [6]
and		
Ganciclovir 7.5–10 mg/kg IV q12 h (for low-level UL97 resistance) [4]		CMX-001, maribavir, leflunomide and artesunate have been used [7,8]
or		Some add CMVIg (e.g. Cytogam 100–150 mg/kg three times per week)
Foscarnet 60 mg/kg q8 h or 90 mg/kg q12 h		Adoptive immunotherapy (infusion of CMV-specific CD8+ T cells) remains experimental
or		
Combined half-dose ganciclovir and half-dose foscarnet [5]		

BID, twice daily; CMV, cytomegalovirus; CMVIg, cytomegalovirus immunoglobulin; IV, intravenous; PO, by mouth.

[a]Oral therapy is not well evaluated in pediatric patients for CMV treatment.

[b]Drug doses: The stated drug doses are for patients with normal renal function. Adjust the drug doses during renal impairment.

- Ganciclovir IV: creatinine clearance (CrCl – ml/min) > 70: 5 mg/kg q12 h; CrCl 50–69: 2.5 mg/kg q12 h; CrCl 25–49: 2.5 mg/kg q24 h; CrCl 10–24: 1.25 mg/kg q24 h; CrCl < 10 or hemodialysis: 1.25 mg/kg three times weekly; continuous renal replacement therapy (CRRT): 2.5 mg/kg q24 h
- Valganciclovir PO: CrCl > 60: 900 mg PO BID; CrCl 40–59: 450 mg BID; CrCl 25–39: 450 mg q24 h; CrCl 10–24: 450 mg q48 h; CrCl < 10 and hemodialysis: not recommended
- Foscarnet: CrCl > 80: 60 mg/kg q8 h or 90 mg/kg q12 h (adjust accordingly for renal function)
- Cidofovir: CrCl > 80: 5 mg/kg weekly for 2 weeks and every 2 weeks thereafter (adjust for renal function; contraindicated if CrCl < 55, proteinuria >100 mg/dL, and serum creatinine >1.5 mg/dL)
- Toxicity: commonly observed toxicities are leukopenia, neutropenia, and suppression of other blood cell lineage (for ganciclovir and valganciclovir); renal toxicities (for foscarnet and cidofovir); electrolyte imbalance particularly with divalent cations (foscarnet) and ocular toxicity (cidofovir).

[c]Foscarnet or cidofovir is generally not used unless resistance is suspected or the patient is intolerant to ganciclovir.

[d]Detectable CMV in the blood by PCR or antigenemia, but without any apparent clinical manifestations.

[e]In all cases, reduction of immunosuppression should be part of CMV management. Monitor for possible allograft rejection if immunosuppression is reduced.

[f]CMV syndrome is defined by the clinical manifestations of fever, myalgias, and bone marrow suppression.

[g]Severity as assessed by the treating clinician, based on the clinical manifestations and the degree of viral load.

References (in square brackets): [1] *Am J Transplantation* 2009; **9**(5): 1205; [2] *Am J Transplantation* 2007; **7**(9): 2106; [3] *Am J Transplantation* 2005; **5**(2): 218; [4] *Transplant Infect Dis* 2008; **10**(2): 129; [5] *Clin Infect Dis* 2002; **34**(10): 1337; [6] *Transplant Infect Dis* 2001; **3**(Suppl 2): 20; [7] *Curr Opin Infect Dis* 2008; **21**(4): 433; [8] *Clin Infect Dis* 2008; **46**(9): 1455.

14.5 Suggested algorithm for the management of ganciclovir (GCV)-resistant CMV infection and disease

Suspect ganciclovir-resistant CMV
Virologic: Rising or unsatisfactory decline in viral load after 2 weeks of treatment, or failure to completely eradicate viremia during treatment
Clinical: Persistence of clinical symptoms

UL97 and UL54 genotypic testing

Symptomatic CMV disease

Reduce immunosuppression

Start empiric therapy:
If high risk of resistance (prolonged ganciclovir use, D+/R−):
Foscarnet
Half-dose foscarnet-half dose ganciclovir combination

If low risk of resistance (R+, no prolonged use of ganciclovir):
High-dose IV ganciclovir up to 10 mg/kg BID
Change oral valganciclovir to IV ganciclovir induction

Consider adjunctive CMV hyperimmune globulin (for D+/R−)

Asymptomatic CMV infection (e.g. symptoms have resolved)

Reduce immunosuppression

Continue IV ganciclovir induction therapy
Change from oral valganciclovir therapy to IV ganciclovir
Consider higher-dose IV ganciclovir up to 10 mg/kg BID

If clinical symptoms develop or recur
If sustained rise in viral load

UL97 mutation only

(No UL97 mutation → IV ganciclovir treatment)

Low-level UL97 mutation (<5X GCV IC50; C592G, A594T, A591V, N597D)
→ high-dose induction ganciclovir treatment → switch to foscarnet if no clinical and virologic response

High-level UL97 mutation (>5X GCV IC50; M460V/I, H520Q, A594V, L595S, C603W) → switch to foscarnet or ganciclovir-foscarnet combination → if no response, repeat UL97 and UL54 genotype assay, and consider alternative or experimental therapies (CMX-001, cidofovir, leflunomide, artesunate, maribavir, switch to sirolimus-containing regimen, adoptive T-cell therapy)

UL54 mutation (usually with UL97 mutation)

UL54 *pol* GCV-CDV mutation → Foscarnet; consider adding CMV Ig

UL54 *pol* FOS-GCV mutation → Cidofovir (if susceptible) or full-dose GCV and foscarnet combination; consider adding adjunctive CMV Ig → if no response, consider alternative or experimental therapies (CMX-001, leflunomide, artesunate, maribavir, adoptive T-cell therapy, switching to sirolimus therapy)

BID, twice daily; CDV, cidofovir; CMV, cytomegalovirus; D+/R−, donor positive/recipient negative; FOS, foscarnet; Ig, immunoglobulin.

15 Epstein-Barr Virus and Post-transplant Lymphoproliferative Disorders

Rebecca Madan & Betsy Herold

15.1 Prevention of Epstein-Barr virus (EBV)-related Post-transplant Lymphoproliferative Disorders (PTLDs)

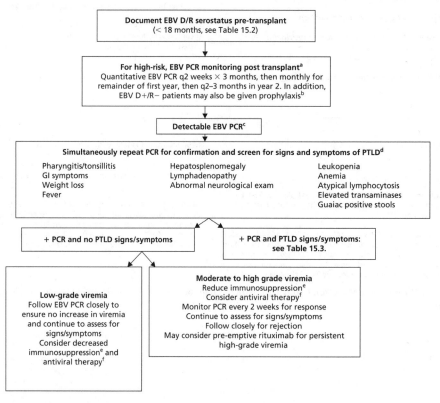

D+/R−, donor positive/recipient negative; PCR, polymerase chain reaction;

[a]High-risk patients are usually EBV D+/R−; EBV D−/R− patients are at risk for community-acquired disease. In some settings, R+ patients may also be at higher risk for PTLD. For D+/R−, resume PCR monitoring every 2 weeks if the patient receives intensification of immunosuppressive therapy for rejection.

[b]In EBV D+/R− patients, some centers use EBV-specific prophylaxis [e.g. valganciclovir (VGCV) or ganciclovir (GCV), same dose as for CMV prophylaxis for 3 months; acyclovir (ACV) or valacyclovir (VACV) are other options] (*Am J Transplantation* 2005; **5**: 2894).

[c]Significant variation between assays and limited data preclude designation of a 'cut-off' for clinically significant viremia. PTLD is often preceded by high-grade viremia, but the positive predictive value of PCR remains low (*Transplant Infect Dis* 2001; **3**: 79). Even low-grade viremia in a previously naïve patient may warrant close monitoring.

[d]The onset of any of these signs/symptoms at any point post-transplant should prompt screening with EBV PCR.

[e]Magnitude and duration of change in immunosuppression are graft- and patient-specific (*Am J Transplantation* 2001; **1**: 103 and *Am J Transplantation* 2005; **5**: 2222).

[f]GCV and ACV have *in vitro* activity against EBV but the role of antivirals in the setting of asymptomatic viremia is unproven. For GCV and VGCV, similar doses as for CMV treatment should be used.

The AST Handbook of Transplant Infections, 1st edition. Edited by D. Kumar & A. Humar. © 2011 Blackwell Publishing Ltd.

15.2 Pediatric EBV serology in donors and recipients < 18 months[a]

Atul Humar

	EBV serology positive	EBV serology negative
Donor < 18 months of age	Assumption = *positive* (even though this may be false positive due to maternal transfer)	Assumption = *negative*
Recipient < 18 months of age	Assumption = *negative* (in this case, assume this is likely due to maternal transfer)	Assumption = *negative*

[a]Serology at < 18 months of age may not be reliable due to passive transfer of antibody. The above assumptions are made to assign the highest risk donor/recipient serostatus to the transplant patient.

15.3 Treatment of PTLD[a]

Rebecca Madan & Betsy Herold

WHO classification of PTLD[b]	Suggested therapy

Early lesions
  Plasmacytic hyperplasia
  Infectious mononucleosis-like
	Reduce immunosuppression[c]
	Consider antiviral therapy[d]
	Rituximab if lesion(s) CD20+ and no response to reduction of immunosuppression

Polymorphic PTLD	Reduce immunosuppression[c] Surgical resection if lesion(s) may result in obstruction Consider antiviral therapy[d] Rituximab (CD20+ lesion) if there is no response to reduction of immunosuppression Consider addition of chemotherapy[f] if no response following rituximab monotherapy

Monomorphic PTLD
B-cell neoplasms
  Diffuse large B-cell lymphoma
  Burkitt/Burkitt-like lymphoma
  Plasma cell myeloma
  Plasmacytoma-like lesion
  Maltoma
  Other
 	
T-cell neoplasma
  Peripheral T-cell lymphoma, not otherwise specified
  Hepatosplenic T-cell lymphoma
  Anaplastic large cell lymphoma
  Natural killer-cell lymphoma
  Other
	Reduce immunosuppression[c]
	Rituximab (CD20+ lesion)[e]
	Chemotherapy[f]
	Surgical resection if lesion(s) may result in obstruction

(Continued)

(*Continued*)

WHO classification of PTLD[b]	Suggested therapy
Hodgkin lymphoma and Hodgkin lymphoma-like PTLD	Reduce immunosuppression[c] Rituximab[e] Chemotherapy[f]

[a]PTLD treatment plans should be patient-specific and formulated by a multidisciplinary team familiar with PTLD management.

[b]Harris NL et al. (2001). PTLD. In: Jaffee ES et al., eds. *Pathology and Genetics: Tumours of Haematopoietic and Lymphoid Tissues (World Health Organization Classification of Tumours)*. Lyons, France: IARC Press, 264.

[c]Where possible, reduction of immunosuppression is important for the treatment of PTLD, although the appropriate magnitude and duration of reduction depends upon multiple factors, including graft type and staging, classification, and aggressiveness of patient's PTLD (*Am J Transplantation* 2001; **1**: 103).

[d]The efficacy of antiviral therapy (acyclovir/ganciclovir) has not been documented by controlled trials. These agents offer the theoretical benefit of preventing spread of lytic phase EBV to previously uninfected B lymphocytes but do not affect the proliferation of EBV-immortalized cells. If used, ganciclovir or vanganciclovir should be given at doses similar to CMV treatment.

[e]Consider initiating rituximab earlier for patients with aggressive lesions or with worsening clinical status on reduced immunosuppression (*Am J Transplantation* 2006; **6**: 569). Rituximab is typically indicated only for lesions with positive CD20 immunostaining.

[f]Chemotherapy regimens are often disease- and patient-specific but may include cyclophosphamide and prednisone therapy (*J Clin Oncol* 2005; **23**: 6481) and combination therapy with cyclophosphamide, doxorubicine, vincristine, and prednisone (CHOP) (*Am J Transplantation* 2006; **6**: 569).

16 Management of herpes simplex virus

Marian G. Michaels

Syndrome	Primary therapy	Alternative therapy	Comments
Primary orolabial/ genital (mucocutaneous) infection	Acyclovir 400 mg PO TID Pediatric dosing (<12 years) : maximum dose is 80 mg/kg/day in three to five divided doses up to 1g/day Acyclovir IV dosing for those unable to tolerate PO therapy: (children and adults) 5–10 mg/kg/dose q8 h	Valacyclovir 1 g PO BID *or* Famciclovir 500 mg PO BID	Therapy is most effective when initiated early in the course of treatment; accordingly it should be started as soon as infection suspected pending viral cultures Most experts recommend continuing treatment until lesions are cleared and for a minimum of five days May switch to oral medication once tolerated Attention to renal function critical particularly when on IV dosing Dosing adjustment with renal impairment may be required
Reactivated orolabial/genital (mucocutaneous) infection	Same as above	Same as above	Same as above
Prevention of reactivation or chronic suppressive therapy	Acyclovir 400–800 mg PO BID Pediatric dosing (<12 years): IV dosing 250 mg/m^2 q8 h *or* Oral dosing 40–80 mg/kg in two to three divided doses up to 1g/day *or* 600 mg/m^2 PO BID	Valacyclovir 500 mg PO BID *or* Famciclovir 250–500 mg PO BID	If the patient is on prophylaxis antiviral medication against CMV (e.g. ganciclovir or valganciclovir) they do not require additional treatment as these medications also offer protection against HSV Many experts recommend prophylaxis against HSV for 1–3 months after transplantation or receipt of rejection therapy in patients who are HSV seropositive Many experts will use suppressive therapy for patients with frequent recurrences of mucocutaneous HSV disease
Keratitis	Topical preparations should be prescribed in conjunction with ophthalmologic evaluation: idoxuridine or vidarabine or trifluridine ± topical steroid	Some experts may add oral treatment in addition to topical	Immediate evaluation by ophthalmologist when HSV keratitis is suspected Acyclovir/valacyclovir/famciclovir PO for prevention may be used

(Continued)

The AST Handbook of Transplant Infections, 1st edition. Edited by D. Kumar & A. Humar. © 2011 Blackwell Publishing Ltd.

(Continued)

Syndrome	Primary therapy	Alternative therapy	Comments
Meningoencephalitis	Acyclovir 10–12.5 mg/kg IV q8h Pediatric dosing: full-term neonates to 12 years of age, 20 mg/kg IV q8h; premature neonates: 20 mg/kg IV q12h	–	Treatment duration 14–21 days Children <3 months should be treated for a minimum of 21 days Many experts recommend repeat evaluation of CSF towards the end of therapy Attention to renal function is critical, particularly when on IV dosing Dosing adjustment with renal impairment may be required
Disseminated disease	Same as above	–	Most experts recommend IV therapy until resolution of disease, then PO therapy can be used except for newborns who should receive a minimum of 21 days of IV treatment Reduce immunosuppression if possible Attention to renal function is critical, particularly when on IV dosing Dosing adjustment with renal impairment may be required
Acyclovir-resistant HSV	Foscarnet IV 80–120 mg/kg/day in two to three divided doses	Cidofovir[a] IV 5 mg/kg once a week × 2 weeks, then q2wk; each dose should be accompanied by probenecid 2 g (per dose) 3 hours prior to cidofovir dose, 1 g (per dose) 1 and 8 hours after completion of the infusion; patients should also receive 1 L of IV normal saline prior to each infusion over 1–2 hours Cidofovir 1% gel for cutaneous lesions (based on availability)	Laboratory confirmation of resistance is recommended although empiric therapy can be started while test results are pending Attention to renal function is critical, particularly when on IV dosing Dosing adjustment with renal impairment is required

BID, twice daily; CMV, cytomegalovirus; CSF, cerebrospinal fluid; IV, intravenous; PO, by mouth; TID, three times daily.
[a]Dosing is based on treatment for CMV

References: [1] *Am J Transplantation* 2009; 9(s4): S104; [2] *MMWR Recomm Rep* 2004; **53**(RR-15): 1; [3] *MMWR Recomm Rep* 2004; **53**(RR-14):1; [4] *MMWR Recomm Rep* 2002; 51(RR-8): 1; [5] *MMWR Recomm Rep* 2000; **49**(RR-10): 1; [6] *Antivir Chem Chemother* 1996; 7: 115.

17 Management of Varicella Zoster Virus

Marian G. Michaels

Syndrome	Primary therapy	Alternative therapy	Prevention	Comments
Primary infection (chickenpox)	Acyclovir IV 10–12.5 mg/kg q8h Pediatric (< 12 years) 500 mg/m²/dose q8h *or* 10 mg/kg/dose q8h	Ganciclovir/ valganciclovir, foscarnet, cidofovir all have activity against VZV but have more toxicity	Prior to transplantation starting at 12 months of age:immunization with varicella vaccine[a]: 0.5 mL SC; a second dose may be administered ⩾ 3 months later For those ≤12 years of age; for those >12 years of age second dose should be given at least 4 weeks after first dose	Some experts recommend using IV therapy for 7–10 days until there are no new lesions for 48 hours Some experts suggest that patients can be changed to oral therapy once they have significantly improved Attention to renal function is critical, particularly when on IV dosing Dosing adjustment with renal impairment may be required Varicella vaccine is a live virus vaccine; while some small studies have documented that it can be used in select circumstances after transplantation, there was a high rate of vaccine-associated rash. Therefore, it is not routinely recommended after transplantation. Every effort should be made to vaccinate prior to transplantation
Disseminated herpes zoster (> one dermatome, non-contiguous) or end-organ disease	Same as above	Same as above	Short-term use of acyclovir PO 600–1000 mg/day divided in three to five doses Pediatric dosing: 250 mg/ m² /dose every 12 hours or valacyclovir 500 mg PO BID	IV treatment should be used until the patient has recovered for a minimum of 7 days but needs to be given longer in those with significant disease or CNS dissemination Attention to renal function is critical, particularly when on IV dosing Dosing adjustment with renal impairment may be required For mild cases, oral therapy (as for local reactivation) can be considered

(Continued)

The AST Handbook of Transplant Infections, 1st edition. Edited by D. Kumar & A. Humar. © 2011 Blackwell Publishing Ltd.

(Continued)

Syndrome	Primary therapy	Alternative therapy	Prevention	Comments
Localized reactivated infection herpes zoster (shingles)	Valacyclovir 1 g PO TID	Acyclovir 800 mg PO five times a day Pediatric dosing (< 12 years of age) 20 mg/kg/dose four times a day (max of 800 mg/dose) *or* Famciclovir 500 mg PO TID	Same as above	
Post-exposure management	Check serostatus in SOT If seropositive SOT: clinically observe If HSCT or sero-negative SOT, then: VariZIG 125 units/10 kg body weight (max 625 units, five vials)	IVIG 400 mg/kg once *or* Acyclovir/valacyclovir/famciclovir[b] PO at the above doses, starting on day 7 after exposure and given for 7 days	Encourage routine immunization of immune-competent people in the community	VZIG is no longer manufactured VariZig or IVIG should be given as soon as possible after exposure and before 96 hours to have the best protective effect

BID, twice daily; CNS, cytomegalovirus; IV, intravenous; PO, by mouth; SC, subcutaneous; SOT, solid organ transplant; TID, three times daily.

[a]Varicella vaccine is not approved for use after transplantation.

[b]Recommended by some experts.

References: [1] *Am J Transplantation* 2009; 9(s4): S108; [2] *Drugs* 1995; 50(2): 396; [3] *MMWR Recomm Rep* 2007; 56(RR-4): 1; [4] National Comprehensive Cancer Network (NCCN) (2008). *Clinical Practice Guidelines in Oncology*™: *Prevention and Treatment of Cancer-Related Infections*, Version 1. NCCN

18 Prevention and Treatment of Human Herpesvirus 6, 7 and 8 Infections in Transplant Recipients

Raymund R. Razonable

	Syndrome	Primary (preferred) Strategy and agent(s)[a]	Alternative strategy and agent(s)[a]	Comments
Prevention				
HHV-6	–	None recommended	None recommended	Antiviral prophylaxis or pre-emptive therapy (monitoring) is not generally recommended for prevention [1]. However, ganciclovir and valganciclovir used for CMV prevention may also prevent HHV-6 reactivation [2]
HHV-7	–	None recommended	None recommended	Antiviral prophylaxis or pre-emptive therapy (monitoring) is not recommended for prevention [1]. Ganciclovir is not active against HHV-7 *in vivo* [2]
HHV-8	–	None recommended	None recommended	Antiviral drugs are not generally recommended for HHV-8 prevention [2]
				Pre-emptive reduction in immunosuppression for high-risk patients and those with detectable HHV-8 viremia [1]
Treatment				
HHV-6	Asymptomatic infection	None recommended	None recommended	Consider reduction in immunosuppression [1]
				The vast majority of HHV-6 infections after solid organ transplant are asymptomatic
				Exclude chromosomally integrated HHV-6 infection (1% of individuals)
	Viral syndrome	Ganciclovir 5 mg/kg IV every 12 hours[b] [3] *or* Valganciclovir 900 mg PO BID *or* Foscarnet IV 60 mg/kg q8 h or 90 mg/kg q12 h	Cidofovir 5 mg/kg weekly for 2 weeks and every 2 weeks thereafter[c]	Reduce immunosuppression[d] Check for CMV co-infection

(*Continued*)

The AST Handbook of Transplant Infections, 1st edition. Edited by D. Kumar & A. Humar. © 2011 Blackwell Publishing Ltd.

(*Continued*)

	Syndrome	Primary (preferred) Strategy and agent(s)[a]	Alternative strategy and agent(s)[a]	Comments
	Tissue-invasive disease (e.g. encephalitis)	Ganciclovir 5 mg/kg IV every 12 hours[b] [3–5] *or* Foscarnet IV 60 mg/kg q8h or 90 mg/kg q12h [4,5]	Cidofovir 5 mg/kg IV weekly for 2 weeks and every 2 weeks thereafter[c]	Reduce immunosuppression Check for CMV co-infection
HHV-7	Asymptomatic infection	None recommended	None recommended	Consider reducing immunosuppression
	Symptomatic infection	Foscarnet IV 60 mg/kg q8h or 90 mg/kg q12h	Cidofovir 5 mg/kg IV weekly for 2 weeks and every 2 weeks thereafter[c]	Reduce immunosuppression Check for CMV co-infection Ganciclovir is not active against HHV-7 *in vivo* based on observational studies [2]
HHV-8	Asymptomatic infection	Reduction in immunosuppression		Consider conversion of immunosuppressive therapy to sirolimus [1]
	Malignant manifestations (e.g. Kaposi's sarcoma)	Reduction in immuno-suppression [1] Conversion of immu-nosuppressive therapy to sirolimus-containing regimen [1] Evaluate for excision surgery, radiation therapy, and chemo-therapy [1]		Antiviral drugs are not effective for malignant HHV-8 disease.

CMV, cytomegalovirus; HHV, human herpesvirus; IV, intravenous; PO, by mouth.

[a]Dosages are those recommended for the treatment of CMV disease. None of these antiviral therapies have been subjected to controlled clinical trials against HHV-6, HHV-7, and HHV-8 infections.

[b]HHV-6 variants A and B have varying ganciclovir susceptibility pattern; HHV-6A is more resistant to ganciclovir [3]. Hence, consider using foscarnet as first-line therapy if specific HHV-6 variant is not known, and if clinical symptoms are severe.

[c]Cidofovir is not a preferred agent due to high risk of renal toxicity.

[d]Reduce immunosuppression: In all cases, reduction of immunosuppression should be part of management if symptoms are present. Monitor for possible allograft rejection if immunosuppression is reduced.

Drug doses: dosages are those recommended for the treatment of CMV disease. None of these antiviral therapies have been subjected to controlled clinical trials against HHV-6, HHV-7, and HHV-8 infections. The drug doses in the table are for patients with normal renal function. Adjust the drug doses during renal impairment:

- Ganciclovir IV: creatinine clearance (CrCl) > 70: 5 mg/kg q12h; CrCl 50–69: 2.5 mg/kg q12h; CrCl 25–49: 2.5 mg/kg q24h; CrCl 10–24: 1.25 mg/kg q24h; CrCl <10 or hemodialysis: 1.25 mg/kg three times weekly; continuous renal replacement therapy (CRRT): 2.5 mg/kg q24h
- Valganciclovir PO: CrCl > 60: 900 mg PO BID; CrCl 40–59: 450 mg BID; CrCl 25–39: 450 mg Q24h; CrCl 10–24: 450 mg q48h; CrCl <10 and hemodialysis: not recommended
- Foscarnet: CrCl > 80: 60 mg/kg q8h or 90 mg/kg q12h (adjust accordingly for renal function)
- Cidofovir: CrCl > 80: 5 mg/kg weekly for 2 weeks and every 2 weeks thereafter (adjust for renal function; contraindicated if CrCl<55, proteinuria > 100 mg/dL, and serum creatinine > 1.5 mg/dl)

References: [1] *Am J Transplantation* 2009; **9**(s4): S97; [2] *J Infect Dis* 2005; **192**(8): 1331; [3] *J Neurovirol* 2006; **12**(4): 284; [4] *Clin Infect Dis* 2002; **34**(3): 309; [5] *Herpes* 2006; **13**(1): 20.

19 BK Polyomavirus and Polyomavirus-associated Nephropathy

Hans H. Hirsch

19.1 Screening, diagnosis and intervention for polyomavirus-associated nephropathy (PyVAN) after renal transplantation

	PyVAN		
	Possible	Presumptive	Definitive
Urine	+	+	+
Decoy cells in urine cytology			
Quantitative BKV RNA in urine			
BKV RNA in urine			
Polyomavirus particles in urine			
Plasma	–	+	+
Quantitative BKV DNA in blood			
Biopsy	–	–	+
Histology			Pattern
Viral cytopathic changes			A
Inflammatory infiltrate			B_1, B_2, B_3
Tubular atrophy/fibrosis			C
Adjunct tools			
Immunohistochemistry			
In situ hybridization			
Electron microscopy			
Intervention indicated	No	(Yes)	Yes

The AST Handbook of Transplant Infections, 1st edition. Edited by D. Kumar & A. Humar. © 2011 Blackwell Publishing Ltd.

19.2 Screening for BK virus (BKV) replication in kidney transplant recipients[a]

Screening/test	Detection	Frequency	Result[b]	Comment
Baseline allograft function				
Urine				
Cytology	Decoy cells	At least every 3 months until 2 years post-transplant	Negative	High negative predictive value for viremia and PyVAN
			Positive	Testing for BKV viremia
Qualitative DNA PCR				Should not be used
Quantitative DNA PCR	BKV large T-antigen (VP1, VP2)	At least every 3 months until 2 years post-transplant	$< 7\log_{10}$geq/mL	No intervention recommended; repeat testing in < 3 months
			$> 7\log_{10}$geq/mL	Testing for BKV viremia
Quantitative RT- PCR	VP1 mRNA	(not defined, consider same as above)	$> 6\log_{10}$copies/ng total RNA	Follow course or consider BKV viremia
Plasma				
Quantitative DNA PCR	BKV large T-antigen (VP1, VP2)	At least monthly until month 3, then every 3 months until 2 years post-transplant	Negative	No intervention recommended
				Repeat testing in 1 month, if viruria is unknown or $>7\log_{10}$geq/mL
			Positive, $< 4\log_{10}$geq/mL	Confirmatory repeat testing within < 1 month
				Some experts recommend adjusting immunosuppression to lower end of target values
				Some experts recommend allograft biopsy
			$> 4\log_{10}$geq/mL	Most experts recommend reducing immunosuppression
				Serum creatinine concentration at least weekly
				Plasma BKV load at least 2-weekly
				Consider allograft biopsy
Impaired function (S-creatinine increasing $> 20\%$ from baseline)				
Plasma				
Quantitative DNA PCR	BKV large T-antigen (VP1, VP2)		Negative	PyVAN unlikely
				No BKV specific intervention recommended
			Positive	No diagnostic thresholds reported Consider kidney biopsy for a definitive diagnosis

(Continued)

Screening/test	Detection	Frequency	Result[b]	Comment
Pediatric recipients Available data suggest earlier and higher incidence of high-level viruria and viremia Better response to treatment, less graft failure		Monthly screening for viruria or viremia until month 6, then 3-monthly until 2 years post-transplant	As above	As above

[a]Adults unless noted otherwise.
[b]Copy number thresholds may vary depending on the assay being used.

19.3 Screening for BKV replication and PyVAN in non-kidney solid organ transplant (SOT) recipients

Screening/test	Target	Frequency	Result	Comment
Baseline allograft function Not generally indicated				BKV viruria is frequent in non-kidney SOT recipients, but BKV viremia and PyVAN are rare
Impaired (S-creatinine increasing > 20% from baseline) Plasma – quantitative DNA PCR	BKV large T-antigen (VP1, VP2)	Definitive PyVAN	Negative	PyVAN in autologous ('native') kidneys is unlikely – no intervention recommended
			Positive	No diagnostic thresholds reported, but most cases $> 4\log_{10}$geq/mL
				Consider kidney biopsy for a definitive diagnosis
			Positive	Most experts recommend reducing immunosuppression (calcineurin inhibitors) to lower range
				Adjunct therapies should be considered, including cidofovir, replacing antimetabolite (e.g. MMF) with leflunomide, and/or mTOR inhibitors, IVIg
				Serum creatinine concentration at least every 2 weeks
				Plasma BKV load at least every 2 weeks

IVIg, intravenous immunoglobulin; MMP, mycophenolate mofetil.

19.4 Treatment of BKV viremia or PyVAN by modification of maintenance immunosuppression

Strategy	Drug	Targets of intervention	Comments
Decreasing	Tac	Trough levels < 6 ng/mL	For PyVAN, often combined with reduction of anti-proliferative drug (Myc or Aza)
	CyA	Trough levels 100–150 ng/mL	For PyVAN, often combined with MMF reduction
	MMF	Dosing 0.5–1 g/day*	For PyVAN, mostly combined with Tac/CyA reduction
Switching	Tac → CyA	Trough levels 100–150 ng/mL	Based on evidence of *in vitro* antiviral activity
			In a case–control study, does not abrogate adverse outcome after late PyVAN diagnosis
	Tac → Sir	Trough levels < 6 ng/mL	Trough levels according to IS protocol employed (dual or triple therapy)
	MMF → Lef	Trough levels 50–100 μg/mL	Based on evidence of *in vitro* antiviral activity of Lef
			Combined with Tac reduction (trough levels ≤ 6 ng/mL)
Discontinuing	MMF/AZA	–	Clinical data for patients with BKV viremia or presumptive PyVAN
			Patients maintained in dual therapy
			As a second step, in patients unresponsive to other approaches
	Tac or CyA	–	Patients on triple Sir/Aza/steroid or Sir/MMF/steroid
Adjunctive therapies	Cidofovir	0.25–1.0 mg/kg q1–2 weeks (efficacy unproven)	Other adjunctive therapies may include IVIg or quinolones (levofloxacin, ciprofloxacin, gatifloxacin), but are unproven
			Modification of immunosuppression remains the mainstay of therapy

AZA, azathioprine; CyA, cyclosporin A; IS, immunosuppression; IVIg, intravenous immuneglobulin; Lef, leflunomide; MMF, mycophenolate mofetil; Myc, mycophenolic acid; Sir, sirolimus; Tac, tacrolimus.

References: [1] *Am J Transplantation* 2009; **9**(s4): S136; [2] *Am J Transplantation* 2007; **7**(12): 2727; [3] *Transplantation* 2008; **85**(12): 1733; [4] *Am J Transplantation* 2010; **10**(2): 407; [5] *Am J Transplantation* 2004; **4**(12): 2082.
*Myfortic MPA equivalent 375–750 mg/day.

20 Respiratory Viruses

Oriol Manuel

20.1 Prevention and treatment of respiratory viral infections after transplantation

Virus/clinical manifestations	Suggested treatment regimens	Prevention	Comments
Adenovirus			
URTI, pneumonia, gastro-enteritis, disseminated infection mostly in pediatric HSCT populations Hemorrhagic cystitis in HSCT	*Primary* In severe pneumonia, cidofovir 5 mg/kg once weekly × 2 weeks, then every 2 weeks (min. four doses) + probenecid or cidofovir 1 mg/kg three times per week In hemorrhagic cystitis intravesical cidofovir (5 mg/kg in 100 mL saline) *Alternative* Ribavirin[a] and ganciclovir have also been used, with discordant results	*Prophylaxis* No data available on efficacy of IVIg *Vaccine* Not available	Efficacy of cidofovir is not proven. Most experience is in HSCT and pediatric lung transplants A multicenter trial using an orally bioavailable lipid conjugate of cidofovir (CMX001) for preemptive treatment of adenovirus viremia in HSCT recipients is ongoing. Response is usually monitored with serial quantitative virology
Bocavirus			
URTI and gastroenteritis	*Primary* None	*Prophylaxis* None *Vaccine* None	Pathogenic role debated
Coronavirus			
URTI and LRTI in HSCT	*Primary* None	*Prophylaxis* None *Vaccine* None	
SARS Coronavirus			
RTI, ARDS in 25% of cases, mortality 9–12%	*Primary* None established	*Prophylaxis* None *Vaccine* None	Ribavirin, interferon-α and corticosteroids were used but considered not effective

(Continued)

The AST Handbook of Transplant Infections, 1st edition. Edited by D. Kumar & A. Humar. © 2011 Blackwell Publishing Ltd.

(Continued)

Virus/clinical manifestations	Suggested treatment regimens	Prevention	Comments
Enteroviruses			
Aseptic meningitis and encephalitis, URTI and LRTI, myocarditis	*Primary* None *Alternative* Consider IVIg 0.5 g/kg for 3–5 days	*Prophylaxis* None *Vaccine* None	Pleconaril is no longer available
Human metapneumovirus			
Acute URTI and LRTI, fatal pneumonia in HSCT	*Primary* None *Alternative* Ribavirin used in case reports Efficacy not proven	*Prophylaxis* None *Vaccine* None	
Measles			
Pneumonia and encephalitis more common in transplant recipients	*Primary* Vitamin A 50 000-200 000 IU OD for two consecutive days in pediatric cases *Alternative* In severe cases ribavirin can be used	*Prophylaxis* Post-exposure prophylaxis with specific immunoglobulin 0.5 mL/kg IM within 6 days of exposure *Vaccine* Two doses of vaccine at least 1 month apart. The vaccine is contraindicated after SOT but may be used in select patients after HSCT (see vaccine section)	–
Parvovirus B19			
Arthritis, aplastic anemia, glomerulonephritis in kidney transplant recipients	*Primary* IVIg 0.4 g/kg for 5 days *Alternative* –	*Prophylaxis* None *Vaccine* None	Consider prolonged therapy with IVIg for persistent replication
Parainfluenzavirus			
URTI and LRTI, croup, asymptomatic infection is common in HSCT recipients	*Primary* None *Alternative* Ribavirin (dose below) for 7–10 days + IVIg 0.5 g/kg for 3–5 days tried with minimal efficacy	*Prophylaxis* None *Vaccine* None	Follow-up of viral load by serial quantitative PCR probably useful for decision to stop treatment

(Continued)

Virus/clinical manifestations	Suggested treatment regimens	Prevention	Comments
Rhinovirus			
Mostly URTI, although can progress to LRTI	*Primary* None	*Prophylaxis* None *Vaccine* None	Pleconaril is no longer available. Role of rhinovirus in development of BOS is more debated than other respiratory viruses
Respiratory syncytial virus			
URTI and LRTI, high mortality described in HSCT and lung transplant recipients	*Primary* Ribavirin (dose below) for 7–10 days + IVIg 0.5 g/kg for 3–5 days, and/or palivizumab 15 mg/kg IV single dose, or RSV Ig (not currently commercially available) *Alternative* Some centers use additional IV methylprednisolone 500 mg daily for 3 days with unclear benefit	*Prophylaxis* Palivizumab 15 mg/kg IV once a month during RSV season in pediatric transplant recipients *Vaccine* None	Follow-up of viral load by serial quantitative PCR probably useful for decision to stop treatment Palivizumab (mAb against RSV gpF) generally used to prevent progression to LRTI Motavizumab (new generation mAb against RSV gpF) is currently under evaluation

ARDS, acute respiratory distress syndrome; BOS, bronchiolitis obliterans syndrome; gpF, glycoprotein F; HSCT, hematopoietic stem cell transplant; IM, intramuscular; IV, intravenous; IVIg, intravenous immunoglobulin; mAb, monoclonal antibody; LRTI, lower respiratory tract infection; OD, once daily; RSV, respiratory syncytial virus; SARS, severe acute respiratory syndrome; URTI, upper respiratory tract infection; SOT, solid organ transplantation.

[a]Dose recommendation for ribavirin (off label use):

- *Intravenous*: 15–25 mg/kg/day in three divided doses every 8 h for 7–10 days. Some authors give a loading dose of 35 mg/kg in three divided doses. There have been some positive experiences with higher doses (60 mg/kg/day in four divided doses).
- *Inhaled*: 6 g/day continuously for 15–18 h/day or 2 g for 1–4 h three times daily.
- *Oral*: 15–25 mg/kg/day in three divided doses for 7–10 days.

Note: intravenous and inhaled ribavirin are not available in most European countries. Ribavirin is associated with dose-dependent hemolytic anemia. In hepatitis C infection, plasma levels of ribavirin $\geq 3 \,\mu g/mL$ have been associated with improved response, but no data exist on respiratory virus infection.

20.2 Prevention and treatment of influenza after transplantation

Influenza virus/clinical manifestations	Suggested treatment regimens[a]	Prevention[a]	Comments
AH1N1, AH3N2, B Influenza in transplant recipients is associated with worse outcome Higher rate of complications (pneumonia, ARDS, obliterative bronchiolitis).	*Primary* Oseltamivir 75 mg BID for 5 days Zanamivir two puffs (10 mg) BID for 5 days (longer duration may be needed; see comments) *Alternative* Amantadine and rimantadine (not useful for 2009 pandemic H1N1, H3N2 and B influenza virus infection)	*Prophylaxis* Oseltamivir 75 mg OD daily or zanamivir two puffs daily for influenza season; because of resistance emergence, post-exposure prophylaxis is not recommended unless started immediately following exposure *Vaccine* Yearly inactivated vaccination for influenza is recommended for all transplant recipients and close contacts	Some authors suggest double dose or extended duration of treatment of oseltamivir (based on *in vitro* data) since viral shedding frequently longer than 5 days IV zanamivir and IV peramivir may be available for compassionate use for severe pneumonia Since 2007–08, a high incidence of oseltamivir-resistant seasonal influenza A H1N1 virus has been found. However, only a few cases of oseltamivir-resistant influenza A H1N1/09 virus have been described. In case of oseltamivir-resistant virus, zanamivir is usually efficacious

ARDS, acute respiratory distress syndrome; BID, twice daily; IV, intravenous; OD, once daily.
[a]Resistance patterns may change and affect recommended antiviral strategies; consult your national health authority regularly for update recommendations.

21 Human Papillomavirus

Gail E. Reid

21.1 Treatment of hand or plantar (cutaneous) warts after transplantation

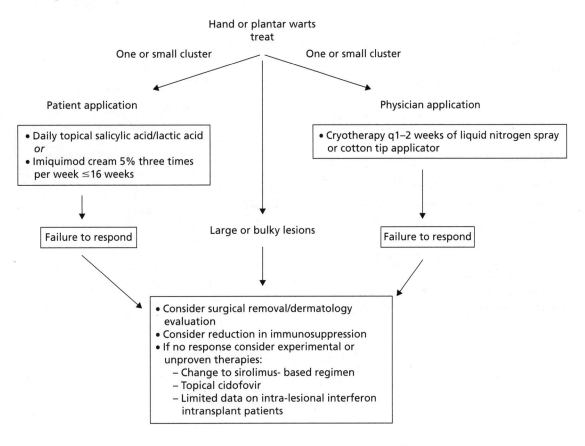

Hand or plantar warts
treat

One or small cluster

One or small cluster

Patient application

Physician application

- Daily topical salicylic acid/lactic acid
  or
- Imiquimod cream 5% three times per week ≤16 weeks

- Cryotherapy q1–2 weeks of liquid nitrogen spray or cotton tip applicator

Failure to respond

Large or bulky lesions

Failure to respond

- Consider surgical removal/dermatology evaluation
- Consider reduction in immunosuppression
- If no response consider experimental or unproven therapies:
  – Change to sirolimus- based regimen
  – Topical cidofovir
  – Limited data on intra-lesional interferon intransplant patients

---

The AST Handbook of Transplant Infections, 1st edition. Edited by D. Kumar & A. Humar. © 2011 Blackwell Publishing Ltd.

21.2 Treatment of external anogenital warts after transplantation

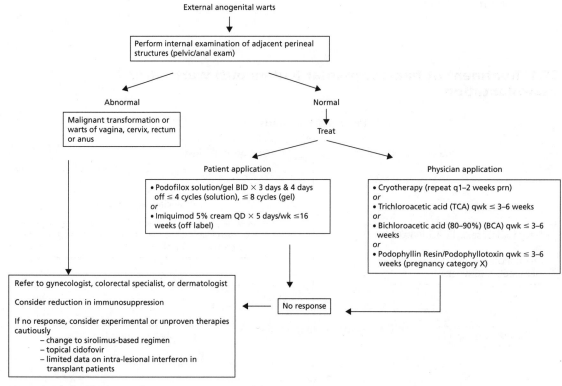

BID, twice daily; QD, once a day.

Reference: *Am J Transplantation* 2009; 9(s4): S151.

22   Hepatitis B

Karen E. Doucette

22.1 Hepatitis B management in hepatitis B surface antigen (HBsAg)-positive recipients

Hepatitis B	
Pre-transplant	Post-transplant
Liver transplant candidate/recipient (HBsAg+)	
Nucleos(t)ide analogue therapy; entecavir 0.5 mg daily or tenofovir 300 mg daily preferred due to high potency, low risk of resistance [1]	Nucleos(t)ide analogue therapy indefinitely; historically lamivudine 100 mg daily has been used successfully (< 10% recurrence combined with HBIg); entecavir 0.5 mg daily or tenofovir 300 mg daily may be preferred due to high potency, low risk of resistance *plus*
Reduction of viral load (undetectable or at least < 2×10^4 IU/mL) reduces risk of post-transplant HBV recurrence	HBIg (IV or IM): the route and doses of HBIg used vary by center and no comparative studies are available. Classic dosing is: 10 000 IU IV during the anhepatic phase of surgery, then 10 000 IU IV daily during the first postoperative week, then according to the anti-HBs blood levels (target value ⩾ 100 IU/L) thereafter
Interferon contraindicated	
	Recently, low-dose HBIg (400-800 IU monthly IM) combined with lamivudine has been shown to result in only 3.4% recurrence in 5 years [2]. In those with undetectable HBV DNA at transplant, discontinuation of HBIG may be considered after 6–12 months [3]
Non-hepatic transplant candidate/recipient (HBsAg+)	
Pre-transplant liver biopsy not routinely required; may be considered if clinically indicated based on published guidelines [1]	Nucleos(t)ide analogue therapy indefinitely [3]. In those with high viral load and/or advanced fibrosis, entecavir 0.5 mg daily or tenofovir 300 mg daily is preferred due to high potency, low risk of resistance
Consideration for therapy should be based on published treatment guidelines; entecavir 0.5 mg daily or tenofovir 300 mg daily is preferred due to high potency, low risk of resistance [1]	In those with low viral load (< 2000 IU/mL) lamivudine 100 mg daily, telbivudine 600 mg daily, or adefovir 10 mg daily are also options
Inactive carriers (HBeAg-negative, normal ALT, HBV DNA < 2000 U/mL) should be monitored off therapy with liver enzymes, liver function tests and HBV DNA every 3–6 months until the time of transplant.	For live donor transplants, initiate antiviral therapy 1 week prior to transplant; for deceased donor transplants, initiate antiviral therapy immediately when donor identified
	Post-transplant monitoring should include liver enzymes, liver function tests and HBV DNA every 3–6 months and abdominal ultrasound every 6–12 months

ALT, alanine transaminase; HBIg, hepatitis B immunoglobulin; HBeAg, hepatitis B e antigen; HBV, hepatitis B virus.
References: [1] *Hepatology* 2009; **50**(3); [2] *Gastroenterology* 2009; **132**; [3] *Am J Transplantation* 2009; **9**(S4).

The AST Handbook of Transplant Infections, 1st edition. Edited by D. Kumar & A. Humar. © 2011 Blackwell Publishing Ltd.

22.2 Hepatitis B management in anti-HBc-positive, HBsAg-negative, anti-HBs-positive or -negative recipients

Hepatitis B	
Pre-transplant	Post-transplant
Liver transplant recipient (anti-HBc+/HBsAg–)	
No additional testing or therapy needed pre-transplant	As source of latent HBV is removed, there is a very low risk of HBV reactivation; no specific prophylaxis or monitoring is required
	If there is an unexplained elevation in liver enzymes, check HBsAg, HBV DNA
Non-hepatic transplant recipient (anti-HBc+/HBsAg–)	
Determine anti-HBs status	Risk of reactivation is low (0–5%) and generally occurs within the first year. Optimal strategy for prevention uncertain
No additional testing or therapy needed pre-transplant	
	In those positive for anti-HBs, post-transplant monitoring of anti-HBs every 3 months may be considered as loss of anti-HBs precedes reactivation
	In those positive for anti-HBc only, options include prophylaxis with lamivudine 100 mg daily × 12 months or periodic monitoring (every 1–3 months) of HBsAg and HBV DNA for the first year

anti-HBc, hepatitis B core antibody; anti-HBs, hepatitis B surface antibody; HBsAg, hepatitis B surface antigen; HBV, hepatitis B virus.

23 Hepatitis C Management in Transplant Candidates and Recipients

Karen E. Doucette

Hepatitis C

Pre-transplant	Post-transplant
Liver transplant candidate/recipient	
Compensated cirrhosis (Child-Pugh class A) Consider therapy with PEG-IFN + ribavirin[a] (note that ribavirin relatively contraindicated if GFR < 50 mL/min)	Recurrence of HCV infection is universal 10–25% develop cirrhosis by 5 years post-transplant. Most centers perform protocol liver biopsies (e.g. every 1–2 years) to monitor for evidence of histological recurrence and reserve HCV therapy for patients who develop biopsy-proven recurrence (grade 3 or stage 1–2 by Metavir) [2]
Decompensated cirrhosis (Child-Pugh class B or C) Therapy is poorly tolerated – it carries a high risk of infectious complications and worsening of liver function and has a low chance of success and is therefore generally contraindicated [1]	In those with histologic recurrence therapy should be initiated with PEG-IFN + ribavirin[a]; overall SVR 27% [3] Pre-emptive therapy is generally not recommend as it is very poorly tolerated and has not been clearly shown to delay onset of recurrence
Non-hepatic transplant candidate/recipient	
Liver biopsy to assess histologic disease should be performed as part of transplant assessment [4]	There are no data to guide optimal post-transplant monitoring. Most centers perform liver enzymes and liver function tests every 3–6 months and ultrasound yearly. Consideration may be given to liver biopsy 3-5 years posttransplant in those who are potential candidates for HCV therapy
Mild disease (Metavir stage F0–F2) may be considered for a trial of therapy with PEG-IFN + ribavirin[a]; if not treated or fails therapy, list for non-hepatic transplant	
Moderate–advanced disease (Metavir Stage F3-F4) – treat for hepatitis C with PEG-IFN ± ribavirin (note that therapy contraindicated in cardiac transplant candidates; ribavirin is relatively contraindicated if GFR < 50 mL/min)	In recipients of life-sustaining (e.g. heart, lung) transplants, interferon-based therapy should be avoided due to risk of rejection
If SVR is achieved, list for transplant; if SVR is not achieved, there is a high risk of end-stage liver disease post-transplant. Options include listing on a case-by-case basis for non-hepatic transplant alone, combined transplant, decline/defer for transplant	In renal transplant recipients, PEG-IFN ± ribavirin may be considered on a case-by-case basis in the setting of significant HCV-related liver or renal disease after weighing potential risks (including rejection) and benefits [4]

GFR, glomerular filtration rate; HCV, hepatitis C virus; PEG-IFN, pegylated interferon; SVR, sustained virologic response.

[a]PEG-IFN and ribavirin dose:
- Genotype 1,4: PEG-IFN-α-2a 180 μg subcutaneously (SC) weekly + ribavirin 1000 mg (<75 kg), 1200 mg (≥75 kg) daily × 48–72 weeks *or* PEG-IFN-α-2b 1.5 μg/kg SC weekly + ribavirin daily based on weight: 800 mg (<65 kg), 1000 mg (66–80 kg), 1200 mg (81–105 kg), 1400 mg (>105 kg) × 48–72 weeks
- Genotype 2,3: PEG-IFN-α-2a 180 μg SC weekly + ribavirin 800 mg daily × 24-48 weeks *or* PEG-IFN-α-2b 1.5 μg/kg SC weekly + ribavirin daily based on weight: 800 mg (<65 kg), 1000 mg (66–80 kg), 1200 mg (81–105 kg), 1400 mg (>105 kg) × 24–48 weeks.

References: *Hepatology* 2005; **42**: 255; [2] *Liver Transplantation* 2003; 9(11): S1; [3] *Am J Transplantation* 2006; **6**: 1586; [4] *Am J Transplantation* 2009; 9(S4).

The AST Handbook of Transplant Infections, 1st edition. Edited by D. Kumar & A. Humar. © 2011 Blackwell Publishing Ltd.

24 Management Algorithm for Transplantation in Patients with Human Immunodeficiency Virus

Shirish Huprikar

24.1 Initial pre-transplant evaluation of patients with human immunodeficiency virus (HIV)

Candidates should undergo a comprehensive evaluation by an HIV specialist with experience in transplant infectious diseases. A detailed history of HIV RNA levels, CD4 cell counts, antiretroviral therapies, resistance testing, and opportunistic infections is essential for identifying appropriate candidates and implementing a comprehensive post-transplant treatment plan to minimize HIV-related complications.

HIV-specific	General
• HIV RNA levels in the past 12 months • Baseline HIV RNA level • CD4 cell counts in the past 12 months • CD4 cell count nadir • Current and previous antiretroviral regimen history • Prior HIV genotypic and phenotypic information • Previous opportunistic infections and treatment history	• Hepatitis A IgG • Hepatitis B: HBsAg, anti-HBs, anti-HBc • Hepatitis C: HCV Ab • HCV RNA, genotype, and treatment history (for HCV Ab+ patients). • HCV RNA and Prior HCV treatment history • Screening for latent TB: TST or IGRA • CMV IgG, EBV IgG, VZV IgG • Syphilis screen • *Strongyloides stercoralis* IgG (for patients who have lived in endemic regions) • *Toxoplasma* IgG • G6PD

Ab, antibody; CMV, cytomegalovirus; G6PD, glucose-6-phosphate dehydrogenase; EBV, Epstein–Barr virus; anti-HBc, hepatitis B core antibody; HBeAg, hepatitis B e antigen; HBsAg, hepatitis B surface antigen; HBV, hepatitis B virus; IGRA, interferon gamma release assays; IgG, immunoglobulin G; TST, tuberculin skin test.

The AST Handbook of Transplant Infections, 1st edition. Edited by D. Kumar & A. Humar. © 2011 Blackwell Publishing Ltd.

24.2 HIV patient selection criteria for transplantation

Suitable candidates for transplantation must adhere to all transplant center-specific selection criteria and have stable HIV.

Organ	HIV RNA	CD4+ T-cell count
Kidney[a]	Undetectable (< 48 copies/mL) for 3 months	> 200 /μL for 3 months
Liver	Undetectable (< 48 copies/mL) for 3 months[b]	> 100 /μL for 3 months in liver candidates without a history of opportunistic infection
		> 200 /μL for 3 months in liver candidates with a history of opportunistic infection

[a]The criteria for kidney candidates should be followed in heart, lung, or pancreas transplant candidates where experience is quite limited.
[b]Detectable HIV RNA is acceptable in selected liver transplant candidates who currently cannot tolerate antiretroviral therapy due to hepatoxicity provided that genotypic testing does not reveal significant resistance that would prevent complete virologic suppression after transplantation.

24.3 Preferred antiretroviral drugs in HIV1 transplant candidates or recipients

Select the simplest and safest regimen that will successfully suppress viremia and maintain CD4 cell counts. Any antiretroviral regimen that consists of preferred or accepted agents and successfully suppresses viremia is appropriate. Long-term non-progressors who achieve undetectable viral loads without antiretrovirals are also acceptable candidates.

Class	Preferred	Alternative	Comments
Dual NRTI	Tenofovir/emtricitabine *or* Abacavir/lamivudine	Zidovudine (avoid in HCV co-infected patients who may need therapy with interferon and ribavirin)	Individual components of fixed-dose combinations need to be administered in patients with renal failure Tenofovir/emtricitabine is preferred in HIV-HBV co-infected patients
NNRTI	Efavirenz	Nevirapine *or* Etravirine	Avoid nevirapine in liver transplant candidates
PI (boosted)	Atazanavir *or* Darunavir	Lopinavir-ritonavir *or* Fos-amprenavir	Decreased levels of atazanavir may occur with gastric acid suppression
Integrase inhibitor	Raltegravir	N/A	–
CCR5 inhibitor	N/A	Maraviroc	–

HBV, hepatitis B virus; HCV, hepatitis C virus; NRTI, nucleoside reverse transcriptase inhibitor; NNRTI, non-nucleoside reverse transcriptase inhibitor; PI, protease inhibitor.

Notes:
- Antiretrovirals that avoid drug interactions with calcineurin inhibitors (CNIs) and sirolimus should be considered to minimize post-transplant complications (see Table 24.4).
  - Raltegravir is a preferred key third agent that avoids drug interactions with CNIs and sirolimus.
  - Efavirenz is a preferred key third agent with limited drug interactions with CNIs and sirolimus (see Table 24.4).
  - Protease inhibitors have significant drug interactions with CNIs and sirolimus. It is reasonable to consider switching the PI to either efavirenz or raltegravir prior to transplantation. The advantage of this approach is to confirm safety, tolerability, and continued virologic suppression prior to transplantation. However, successful switches to raltegravir in the post-transplant setting have been described without complications.
- For living donor transplant recipients, one may consider initiating the CNI or sirolimus prior to transplantation in the setting of PIs to achieve therapeutic levels at the time of transplantation and avoid sub-therapeutic or toxic levels in the early post-transplant period.
- HBV co-infected patients should have HBV DNA levels suppressed prior to transplantation. This can usually be achieved by selecting an antiretroviral regimen than includes at least one (ideally two) drug(s) with activity against HBV. Lamivudine, emtricitabine, and tenofovir all have activity against both HIV and HBV. The fixed-dose combination of emtricitabine and tenofovir all is the ideal NRTI backbone for the HIV-HBV co-infected patient with normal renal function. If necessary, entecavir or adefovir can be added to the antiretroviral regimen to control HBV.
- HCV co-infected non-liver transplant candidates must undergo a thorough evaluation that includes liver biopsy. Patients without cirrhosis should be evaluated for therapy with pegylated interferon and ribavirin prior to transplantation with the goal of achieving a sustained virologic response prior to transplantation as HCV can progress more rapidly in the setting of post-transplant immunosuppression and interferon is relatively contraindicated following renal transplantation.
- Update immunizations pre-transplant: inactivated influenza (annually), pneumococcal polysaccharide vaccine, hepatitis A, hepatitis B, diphtheria, tetanus and polio (DTaP).

24.4 Drug–drug interactions and post-transplant management in transplanted patients with HIV

Post-transplant antibody induction therapy is generally avoided in this subset of patients due to an increased risk of serious bacterial infections.

Antiretroviral(s)	Potential interaction	Approximate dosing adjustment	CNI/sirolimus serum levels
Ritonavir-boosted PIs Nelfinavir	Increased levels of CNI or sirolimus	Tacrolimus 0.5–1.5 mg weekly Cyclosporine 25–50 mg daily Sirolimus 1–1.5 mg weekly	Early and frequent monitoring are required to establish dose and frequency
Unboosted PIs Atazanavir Fos-amprenavir	Increased levels of CNI or sirolimus	Tacrolimus 0.5–1.5 mg weekly Cyclosporine 100–200 mg daily Sirolimus 1–1.5 mg daily	Early and frequent monitoring are required to establish dose and frequency
NNRTI (efavirenz, nevirapine, etravirine)	Decreased levels of CNI or sirolimus	No baseline adjustments	Early monitoring is needed as higher doses may be required
NNRTI + PI	Increased levels of CNI or sirolimus	Tacrolimus 0.5–1.5 mg weekly Cyclosporine 25–50 mg daily Sirolimus 1 mg weekly	Early and frequent monitoring are required to establish dose and frequency
Integrase inhibitor (ralregravir)	None	No dose adjustment	Standard monitoring
CCR5 inhibitor (maraviroc)	May increase maraviroc levels	No dose adjustment	Standard monitoring

CNI, calcineurin inhibitor; HBV, hepatitis B virus; HCV, hepatitis C virus; NRTI, nucleoside reverse transcriptase inhibitor; NNRTI, non-nucleoside reverse transcriptase inhibitor; PI, protease inhibitor.
Notes:
- Pharmacokinetic studies evaluating relatively newer PIs (e.g. atazanavir, darunavir) and the second-generation NNRTI (etravirine) are needed. Until then, clinicians should assume similar interactions and dose CNIs and sirolimus accordingly.
- One of the following approaches for re-initiating antiretrovirals (ARVs) post-transplant should be considered:
  - Re-introduce ARVs only after patients and graft function have stabilized. The rationale of this approach is to avoid direct ARV toxicity in the graft as well as the challenging drug interactions in the early transplant period. CNI or sirolimus should be held on the day (or perhaps the day before) the PI-containing ARV regimen is resumed. Daily levels of CNI or sirolimus should be monitored to guide dosing. CNI or sirolimus dosing should be avoided on the day after starting a boosted PI even if the level is within the therapeutic window, as serum levels can continue to rise in the setting of a boosted PI before they fall.
  - Immediately resume ARVs concurrently with immunosuppressants when the patient is tolerating oral medications. The rationale of this approach is to maintain virologic suppression in the early post-transplant period and prevent the risks associated with reduced cellular immune function. A single dose of the CNI or sirolimus should be given in patients on PI-containing regimens followed by daily levels to guide the appropriate dose and interval.
- HIV RNA levels and CD4 counts should be monitored at least every 3 months.
- Pneumocystis pneumonia prophylaxis should be continued indefinitely.
- Secondary prophylaxis should be considered in patients with a prior history of an OI.
- All other standard Opportunistic infection prevention strategies should be followed.
- Serial liver biopsy should be considered in HCV co-infected liver transplant recipients due to a greater risk for early HCV recurrence.

References: [1] *J Am Med Assoc* 2010; **304**(3):321; [2] *Rev Med Virol* 2009; **19**(6): 317; [3] http://hivinsite.ucsf.edu/insite?page=ar-00-02&post=10&param=19; [4]*Am J Transplantation* 2007; **7**(12): 2816; [5] *Am J Transplantation* 2009; **9**(8): 1946; [6] *Am J Transplantation* 2006; **6**(4): 753.

25 Management of Selected Fungal Infections After Transplantation

Michele I. Morris

25.1 Management of selected fungal infections after transplantation

Fungal infection	Treatment / alternative therapy	Prophylaxis	Comments
Candidiasis (*C. albicans, C. glabrata, C. tropicals, C. parapsilosis, C. krusei* and others)			
Thrush	Fluconazole 100–200 mg PO daily *Alternative therapy* Clotrimazole troches 10 mg PO five times daily, nystatin suspension 5–10 mL swish or pastilles PO QID	Liver, intestinal, or pancreas: fluconazole 200–400 mg IV/PO daily × 4–10 weeks. Often used only if there are risk factors *or* Echinocandin[a] *or* L-AmB products[a]	*C. krusei* is resistant to fluconazole. *C. glabrata* may become azole-resistant. For *C. parapsilosis*, fluconazole is preferred over echinocandin Susceptibility testing is recommended for all sterile-site isolates
Esophageal	Fluconazole 200–400 mg PO daily *or* Caspofungin 70 mg IV load, then 50 mg IV daily or micafungin 150 mg IV daily or anidulafungin 200 mg IV load then 100 mg IV daily × 7–14 days *Alternative therapy* Voriconazole 200 mg PO BID *or* Posaconazole 400 mg PO BID *or* ABLC or L-AmB 3 mg/kg/day × 7–14 days		Drug interactions between azoles and CNI (see Chapter 53) Caution is needed with IV voriconazole in renal dysfunction For bone, joint, or heart valve infections, there are limited data on echinocandins. Use azole or a lipid amphotericin product

(Continued)

The AST Handbook of Transplant Infections, 1st edition. Edited by D. Kumar & A. Humar. © 2011 Blackwell Publishing Ltd.

Fungal infection	Treatment/ alternative therapy	Prophylaxis	Comments
UTI	Fluconazole 200–400 mg PO/IV daily *Alternative therapy* Lipid amphotericin product 3 mg/kg/day or Echinocandin (poor urinary levels, see comments)		For fluconazole-resistant UTI: caspofungin 70 mg IV × one dose, then 50 mg IV daily (poor urine levels but small case series). Voriconazole achieves poor urinary levels Amphotericin bladder washes may be used, although efficacy is unclear
Invasive (fungemia, abscess, peritonitis, hepatosplenic)	Caspofungin 70 mg IV load, then 50 mg IV daily or micafungin 100 mg IV daily or anidulafungin 200 mg IV load, then 100 mg IV daily) or Fluconazole 400–800 mg IV daily (only for fluconazole-sensitive *Candida*) *Alternative therapy* ABLC 5 mg/kg/day or L-AmB 5 mg/kg/day or Voriconazole 6 mg/kg IV × two doses, then 4 mg/kg IV q12 h		
Aspergillosis – invasive pulmonary aspergillosis, sinusitis, cerebral aspergillosis, disseminated disease (*A. fumigatus*, *A. flavus*, *A. niger*, *A. terreus*)	Voriconazole 6 mg/kg IV q12 h × two doses, then 4 mg/kg IV q12 h or Combination therapy with voriconazole + echinocandin (caspofungin, micafungin, or anidulafungin) *Alternative therapy* ABLC 5 mg/kg/day or L-AmB 3–5 mg/kg/day or Posaconazole 200 mg PO QID till response, then 400 mg PO BID Note: *A. terreus* is resistant to amphotericin products	Lung: voriconazole 200 mg PO BID × 3–6 months or Itraconazole 200 mg PO BID or Inhaled AmBd, inhaled ABLC, inhaled L-AmB (doses vary, see Tables 11 and 40) Liver/intestinal/multivisceral: echinocandin or L-AmB 3–5 mg/kg/day for 2–4 weeks Heart: voriconazole 200 mg PO BID or itraconazole 200 mg PO BID × 50–150 days	Consider combination therapy for moderate to severe disease There is significant drug interaction of voriconazole and CNIs. CNI dose reduction is indicated. Drug interactions (see Chapter 53)

(Continued)

(*Continued*)

Fungal infection	Treatment/ alternative therapy	Prophylaxis	Comments
Cryptococcosis meningitis, brain abscess, pneumonia, lung nodule, disseminated (*Cryptococcus neoformans* or *C. gattii*)	For CNS disease: (ABLC 5 mg/kg/day *or* L-AmB 3–5 mg/kg/day) ±5-flucytosine 150 mg/kg/day divided q6h followed by fluconazole 400–800 mg daily *Alternative therapy* For non-CNS disease: fluconazole 400 mg daily × 6–12 months		Fluconazole 200 mg daily should be used as maintenance therapy after treatment of CNS disease × 6–12 months Drug interactions (see Chapter 53) Immune reconstitution inflammatory syndrome may occur after starting treatment
Histoplasmosis – pulmonary, disseminated (*Histoplasma capsulatum*)	ABLC 5 mg/kg/day *or* L-AmB 3–5 mg/kg/day followed by itraconazole 200 mg PO BID × 1 year minimum *Alternative therapy* Itraconazole 200 mg PO BID (milder cases)	Not defined. Antifungal prophylaxis could be considered in select settings: itraconazole 200 mg PO once daily to BID	Voriconazole and Posaconazole have been used in small numbers of patients with response. Drug interactions (see Chapter 53).
Blastomycosis pulmonary, bone and joint, disseminated (*Blastomyces dermatitidis*)	ABLC 5 mg/kg/day *or* L-AmB 3–5 mg/kg/day followed by itraconazole 200 mg PO BID × 6–12 months minimum *Alternative therapy* Itraconazole 200 mg PO BID (milder cases)	No data	Voriconazole has been used in small numbers of patients with response Drug interactions (see Chapter 53).
Coccidiomycosis – pulmonary, meningitis, bone and joint, disseminated (*Coccidioides immitis*)	ABLC 5 mg/kg/day *or* L-AmB 3–5 mg/kg/day *or* Fluconazole 400 mg daily (for mild to moderate pulmonary disease only) *or* First line for meningitis is fluconazole 400–800 mg daily *Alternative therapy* Itraconazole 200 mg PO BID	If there is a past history of infection or positive serologies, give fluconazole 200–400 mg IV/PO daily. Same regimen for active infection/positive serologies in organ donor. Duration is undefined and may be indefinite	Lifelong suppression with fluconazole especially for meningitis If using ABLC or L-AmB, give for 2–4 weeks, then switch to fluconazole Drug interactions (see Chapter 53).

(*Continued*)

Fungal infection	Treatment/ alternative therapy	Prophylaxis	Comments
Zygomycosis – sinusitis, rhinocerebral, Pulmonary, skin and soft tissue, disseminated (*Mucor, Absidia, Rhizomucor, Rhizopus* and others)	L-AmB 5–10 mg/kg/day *Alternative therapy* Posaconazole 200 mg PO QID until disease is stable, then 400 mg PO BID with fatty meal or Combination therapy (e.g. lipid amphotericin product + posaconazole)	Consider posaconazole 400 mg PO BID in select situations (e.g. acute leukemia, chronic GVHD, secondary prophylaxis, pre-lung transplant colonized)	Consider surgical resection as adjunctive therapy Drug interactions with posaconazole and CNI (see Chapter 53) Combination therapy with caspofungin has also been used ABLC may be less effective than L-AmB Consider G-CSF / GM-CSF
Fusariosis – cutaneous, sinusitis, pulmonary, disseminated (*Fusarium solani, F. oxysporum* and others)	Voriconazole 6 mg/kg IV q12h × two doses, then 4 mg/kg IV q12h or Posaconazole 400 mg PO BID or 200 mg PO QID *Alternative therapy* ABLC 5–10 mg/kg/day or L-AmB 5–10 mg/kg/day		Fusarium species generally more drug-resistant Surgical debridement of localized disease *F. solani* is generally resistant to azoles Remove catheter for catheter-related infections] Drug interactions (see Chapter 53)
Scedosporium – sinusitis, skin and soft tissue, pulmonary, disseminated (*S. apiospermum, S. prolificans*)	Voriconazole 6 mg/kg IV q12h × two doses, then 4 mg/kg IV q12h *S. prolificans* is resistant to all antifungals (see comments) *Alternative therapy* Posaconazole 400 mg PO BID or 200 mg PO QID		Consider surgical debridement for adjunct therapy For *S. prolificans*, consider combination therapy (e.g. voriconazole + terbinafine or itraconazole + terbinafine) Drug interactions (see Chapter 53)
Sporotrichosis (*Sporothrix schenkii*)			
Lymphocutaneous	Itraconazole 200–400 mg PO daily × 3–6 months or until total resolution of all lesions *Alternative therapy* Lymphocutaneous: terbinafine 500 mg PO BID or saturated solution of potassium iodide (SSKI) increasing dose of five to 50 drops TID as tolerated ± 3–6 months		Newer azoles not studied for this infection Consider surgical resection for localized, unresponsive disease Drug interactions (see Chapter 53)

(*Continued*)

(Continued)

Fungal infection	Treatment/ alternative therapy	Prophylaxis	Comments
Invasive (bone, joint, pulmonary, CNS or other)	ABLC 5 mg/kg/day *or* L-AmB 3–5 mg/kg/day followed by itraconazole 200 mg PO BID *Alternative therapy* May consider combination therapy e.g. adding terbinafine 500 mg PO BID		
Dematiaceous fungi skin and soft tissue, sinusitis, pulmonary, disseminated (*Alternaria, Bipolaris, Curvularia* and others)	Itraconazole 200 mg PO BID *Alternative therapy* ABLC 5 mg/kg/day *or* L-AmB 3–5 mg/kg/day *or* Voriconazole 200 mg PO BID		Consider surgical debridement for adjunct therapy Drug interactions between azoles and CNI (see Chapter 53)

AmBd, amphotericin B deoxycholate; ABLC, amphotericin B lipid complex; CNI, calcineurin-inhibitors; CNS, central nervous system; G-CSF, granulocyte colony-stimulating factor; GM-CSF, granulocyte/macrophage colony stimulating factor; GVHD, graft-versus-host disease; IV, intravenous; L-AmB, liposomal amphotericin B; PO, by mouth; QID, three times daily; UTI, urinary tract infection.

[a]Especially if there is a risk of *Aspergillus* or non-*albicans Candida* infection.

References: [1] *Am J Transplantation* 2009; **9**(s4): S192. [2] *Am J Transplantation* 2009; **9**(s4): 208. [3] *Am J Transplantation* 2009; **9**(s4):S180. [4] *Antimicrob Agents Chemother* 2009; **53**(4):1648. [5] *Clin Infect Dis* 2008; **47**(3): 364.

26 Treatment of *Nocardia* Infections

Nina M. Clark

Site of infection	Primary[a,b]	Alternative agents[a,b]	Comments
Pulmonary – mild to moderate[c]	TMP-SMX[d] 15mg/kg/day in two to four divided doses, IV or PO	Imipenem IV 500 mg q6h + amikacin IV 10–15mg/kg/day *or* Minocycline PO/IV 200 mg q12h *or* Linezolid PO/IV 600 mg q12h	Agents such as amoxicillin-clavulanate and fluoroquinolones may be effective but there are few data to support their use as initial therapy; linezolid has excellent activity against all species of *Nocardia* Treat pneumonia for 6–12 months
Pulmonary – severe[c,e]	Imipenem IV 500 mg q6h + amikacin 10–15 mg/kg/day *and/or* TMP-SMX IV 15 mg/kg/day in two to four divided doses	Linezolid IV 600 mg q12h	Use of amikacin may be limited by nephrotoxicity
Cerebral[e]	Imipenem + amikacin *or* TMP-SMX (see doses above)	Linezolid *or* Ceftriaxone IV 2g q12h or Cefotaxime IV 2g q8h *or* Minocycline (see doses above)	Meropenem IV 1g q8h has been used successfully as an alternative to imipenem for brain abscess; ertapenem is not as active *in vitro* Parenteral therapy for 3–6 weeks, then switch to oral therapy; treat for 9–12 months
Disseminated[e]	Imipenem + amikacin or TMP-SMX (see doses above)	Ceftriaxone, cefotaxime, linezolid or minocycline (see doses above)	

IV, intravenous; PO, by mouth; TMP-SMX, trimethoprom- sulfamethoxazole.

[a]No comparative controlled clinical trials are available for therapeutic agents; adjust dosing of antimicrobials as necessary according to renal function.

[b]*Nocardia farcinica*, *N. nova* and *N. otitidiscaviarum* may be resistant to sulfonamides, *N. brasiliensis* is often resistant to imipenem, and *N. farcinica*, *N. transvalensis* and *N. otitidiscaviarum* display resistance to cephalosporins; antimicrobial susceptibility testing is strongly recommended, particularly when treating non-*asteroides Nocardia* or when using alternative regimens.

[c]Investigation should be performed to exclude disseminated disease, including cerebral abscess.

[d]TMP-SMX: sulfonamides such as sulfadiazine (1.5 g four times a day, QID) or sulfisoxazone (2 g QID) may be substituted for TMP-SMX.

[e]A three-drug regimen of imipenem + amikacin + TMP-SMX is recommended by some experts as initial therapy for critically ill patients pending susceptibility testing.

References: [1] *Am J Transplantation* 2009; **9**(s4): S70; [2] *Medicine* 2009; **88**: 250; [3] *Antimicrob Agents Chemother* 2007; **51**: 1102; [4] *Clin Microbiol Rev* 2006; **19**: 259; [5] *Ann Pharmacother* 2007; **41**: 1694.

The AST Handbook of Transplant Infections, 1st edition. Edited by D. Kumar & A. Humar. © 2011 Blackwell Publishing Ltd.

27 Tuberculosis: Treatment and Prevention

Nina M. Clark

27.1 Treatment of latent *Mycobacterium tuberculosis* (TB) infection[a]

Setting of infection	Primary	Alternative agents	Comments
Pre-transplant candidate with latent TB and no prior adequate treatment[b] (assumes INH susceptibility)			
Adults	INH PO 5 mg/kg/day (max. 300 mg/day) for 9 months[c]	INH 15 mg/kg twice weekly by DOT (max. 900 mg/dose) for 9 months	Administer pyridoxine 25–50 mg/day with INH
		RIF 10 mg/kg/day (max. 600 mg/day) for 4 months	INH daily for 6 months not advised as a 9-month course is more efficacious
		Levofloxacin + ethambutol or moxifloxacin + ethambutol for 6 months could be considered if INH and RIF are not tolerated (animal data)	Low risk of hepatotoxicity seen with INH in persons with compensated liver disease awaiting liver transplantation, although many experts recommend delaying treatment until after liver transplant
Children	INH 10–15 mg/kg/day (max. 300 mg/day) for 9 months	INH 20–25 mg/kg twice weekly by DOT for 9 months	Children weighing > 40 kg should be dosed as adults
		RIF 10–20 mg/kg/day (max. 600 mg/day) × 4 months	Organ transplantation may be performed in patients on treatment for latent TB with continuation of therapy after transplant until completion
Post-transplant recipient with latent TB not treated pre-transplant[b]			
Adults	INH 5 mg/kg/day (max. 300 mg/day) for 9 months	INH 15 mg/kg twice weekly by DOT (max. 900 mg/dose) for 9 months	Administer pyridoxine 25–50 mg/day with INH
		Quinolone + ethambutol could be considered (see above)	INH daily for 6 months is not advised due to increased efficacy of 9-month course

(Continued)

The AST Handbook of Transplant Infections, 1st edition. Edited by D. Kumar & A. Humar. © 2011 Blackwell Publishing Ltd.

Setting of infection	Primary	Alternative agents	Comments
Children	INH 10–15 mg/kg/day (max. 300 mg/day) for 9 months	INH 20–25 mg/kg twice weekly by DOT for 9 months	Children weighing > 40 kg should be dosed as adults
			Avoid RIF due to drug interactions with immunosuppressive medications[d]

DOT, directly observed therapy; INH, isoniazid; RIF, rifampin.

[a]All transplant candidates as well as living donors should be assessed for exposure to TB by history and tuberculin skin testing (TST) or interferon-gamma release assays (IGRAs). Some recommend two-step TST.

[b]A positive TST for a transplant recipient is ⩾ 5 mm of induration at 48–72h. Some experts advocate treatment for latent TB in TST-negative individuals with radiographic evidence of prior untreated TB or who have been in recent close contact with a person with active TB. For donor TB issues (see Chapter 39).

[c]Routine laboratory monitoring is recommended for those with abnormal baseline liver function tests and others at risk for hepatic disease; consider testing at 2-week intervals for the first 6 weeks of therapy, then monthly. All those on treatment should be monitored for side-effects monthly. Transaminase elevation of three to five times the upper limit of normal should prompt discontinuation of INH.

[d]RIF is a potent inducer of the metabolism of cyclosporine, tacrolimus and sirolimus and it may be difficult to maintain adequate levels of these immunosuppressives.

27.2 Treatment of active *Mycobacterium tuberculosis* infection

Site of infection/ condition	Primary		Alternative agents	Comments
	Initial phase[b]	Continuation phase[c]		
Pulmonary[a]				
Adults	INH 5 mg/kg/day (max. 300 mg/day) + Rifabutin[d] 5 mg/kg/day (max. 300 mg/day) + ETH[e] 15–25 mg/kg/day (max. 1.6 g/day) + PZA 25–30 mg/kg/day (max. 2 g/day)	INH + rifabutin for 4 months[f]	Levofloxacin PO/IV 1000 mg/day	Administer pyridoxine 50 mg/day with INH
			RIF (see comment)	RIF 10 mg/kg/day (max. 600 mg/day) is part of the standard regimen but is difficult to use in transplant patients due to drug interactions. Rifabutin has fewer drug interactions
			SM 15 mg/kg/day IM or IV (max. 1 g)	
			Second-line agents: KAN 15 mg/kg/day IM or IV (max. 1 g); AMIK 15 mg/kg/day (max. 1 g/day) IM or IV; ethionamide 15–20 mg/kg/day (max. 1 g); cycloserine 10–15 mg/kg/day (max. 1 g) in two divided doses; capreomycin 15 mg/kg/day (max. 1 g IM or IV)	Prolonged aminoglycoside therapy is poorly tolerated in transplant patients
				Daily rather than intermittent dosing is recommended due to risk of relapse and potentially severe fluctuations in immunosuppressive levels with intermittent dosing
				DOT therapy is recommended, as it improves adherence and outcome

(*Continued*)

(Continued)

Site of infection/ condition	Primary		Alternative agents	Comments
	Initial phase[b]	Continuation phase[c]		
Children	INH 10–15 mg/kg/day (max. 300 mg/day) + rifabutin 5 mg/kg/day (max. 300 mg/day) + ETH[e] 15–20 mg/kg/day (max. 1 g/day) + PZA 20–30 mg/kg/day (max. 2 g/day)	INH + rifabutin for 4 months[f]	RIF (see comment) SM 20–30 mg/kg/day IM or IV (max. 1 g) Second-line agents: KAN or AMIK 15–30 mg/kg/day IM or IV (max. 1 g); ethionamide 15–20 mg/kg/day (max. 1 g); cycloserine 15–20 mg/kg/day (max. 1 g) in two divided doses; capreomycin 15–30 mg/kg/day (max. 1 g IM or IV)	Children weighing > 40 kg should be dosed as adults
Central nervous system	Same as for pulmonary	Same regimen as for pulmonary but extend continuation phase to 7–10 months	–	–
Disseminated or bone and joint disease	Same as for pulmonary	Same regimen as for pulmonary but extend continuation phase up to 7 months	–	–
INH resistance	Rifabutin + ETH + PZA ± FQ for 6 months	Not applicable	–	FQ may enhance the treatment efficacy
RIF/rifabutin resistance	INH + ETH + FQ + PZA ± SM or KAN or AMIK	INH + ETH + FQ for 10–16 months	–	–

AMIK, amikacin; DOT, directly observed therapy; ETH, ethambutol; FQ, fluoroquinolone; INH, isoniazid; KAN, kanamycin; PZA, pyrazinamide; RIF, rifampin; SM, streptomycin.

[a]Assumes INH/RIF susceptibility and normal renal function. For multidrug-resistant TB (resistance to two or more drugs including INH and RIF) or extensively drug-resistant TB (resistance to INH, RIF, any FQ and one of KAN, AMIK, or capreomycin), seek expert guidance on recommended treatment.

[b]Initial phase = first 2 months of therapy.

[c]Continuation phase = treatment after initial 2 months of therapy.

[d]Despite drug interactions between rifabutin or RIF and immunosuppressives such as cyclosporine, tacrolimus and sirolimus, a regimen containing one of these drugs is preferred due to its potent activity against TB. Rifabutin is suggested to minimize drug interactions (see 'Comments'). Closely monitor immunosuppressive levels with the use of RIF or rifabutin; higher doses of immunosuppressives are often required.

[e]ETH can be discontinued before 2 months of therapy if TB isolate displays no drug resistance.

[f]If cavitary TB and sputum is still culture-positive at 2 months, extend continuation phase to 7 months.

References: [1] *Am J Transplantation* 2009; **9**(s4): S57; [2] *Am J Respir Crit Care Med* 2003; **167**: 603; [3] *Clin Infect Dis* 2009; **49**: 1276; [4] *Am J Respir Crit Care Med* 2005; **172**(9): 1169; [5] *MMWR* 2005; **54**: 49; [6] *Am J Transplantation* 2007; **7**: 2797; [7] *Am J Respir Crit Care Med* 2005; **172**: 1452.

28 Treatment of Non-tuberculous *Mycobacterium* Infections

Nina M. Clark

Organism[a]	Primary[b,c,d,e]	Alternative agents[b,c,d,e]	Comments
M. avium-intracellulare complex (MAC)	AZ PO 250-500 mg/day + rifabutin PO 300 mg/day + ETH PO 15 mg/kg/day	RIF[f] 600 mg/day; CLARI 500 mg BID; AMIK 10–12 mg/kg/dose three times weekly IM or IV; SM 0.5–1.0 g IV/IM three times weekly; moxifloxacin 400 mg/day	Test isolate for CLARI susceptibility Addition of aminoglycoside three times a week may enhance the efficacy of treatment, although nephrotoxicity may occur Can consider three times weekly administration of AZ (600 mg), CLARI (1000 mg), ETH (25 mg/kg) or rifabutin (300–600 mg) if there is no cavitary disease and if disease is not severe; however, it could cause significant variation in calcineurin inhibitor levels depending on the agent used
M. kansasii	INH PO 5 mg/kg/day (max. 300 mg/day) + rifabutin PO 300 mg/day + ETH PO 15 mg/kg/day	RIF, CLARI, AZ, AMIK, SM, moxifloxacin, SMX 1 g q8–12 h or TMP/SMX	Test for RIF susceptibility; if RIF-resistant, test additional agents; INH may be active even if there is *in vitro* resistance All isolates are resistant to pyrazinamide Give pyridoxine 50 mg daily when using INH
M. abscessus[c]	Base on susceptibility testing Common regimens include AZ + one or two injectable agents	AZ, CLARI, AMIK, cefoxitin IV 8–12 g/day in divided doses, linezolid IV/PO 600 mg q12 h imipenem IV 500 mg q6h, TIG IV 100 mg × 1 then 50 mg q12h	*M. abscessus* lung disease is difficult to cure Injectable agents used for initial 2–6 weeks until improvement Consider surgical debridement
M. chelonae[c]	Base on susceptibility testing, two drugs recommended Common regimens include AZ + another agent	CLARI, AZ, linezolid, tobramycin IV/IM 5 mg/kg/day, imipenem, TIG (see above for doses)	Consider surgical debridement

(Continued)

The AST Handbook of Transplant Infections, 1st edition. Edited by D. Kumar & A. Humar. © 2011 Blackwell Publishing Ltd.

(*Continued*)

Organism[a]	Primary[b,c,d,e]	Alternative agents[b,c,d,e]	Comments
M. fortuitum[c]	Base on susceptibility testing, two drugs recommended	CLARI, AZ, levofloxacin 500–750 mg/day, moxifloxacin, doxycycline PO 100 mg BID, minocycline 100 mg BID, SMX or TMP/SMX, AMIK, imipenem, TIG	Inducible resistance to macrolides – use with caution
M. haemophilum	AZ 250–500 mg/day + rifabutin 300 mg/day + ciprofloxacin 500–750 mg BID	CLARI, RIF, doxycycline, SMX or TMP/SMX	No standardized susceptibility methods. Requires growth temperature of 28–30°C and supplemental media for isolation
M. marinum	AZ 250–500 mg/day + ETH 15 mg/kg/day ± rifabutin 300 mg/day for extensive disease	RIF, CLARI, SMX or TMP/SMX, minocycline, doxycycline	Consider surgical debridement, especially for closed spaces of the hand

AMIK, amikacin; AZ, azithromycin; BID, twice daily; CLARI, clarithromycin; ETH, ethambutol; IM, intramuscular; INH, isoniazid; IV, intravenous; PO, by mouth; RIF, rifampin; SM, streptomycin; SMX, sulfamethoxazole; TIG, tigecycline; TMP, trimethoprim.

[a]See Griffith *et al.* [2] for criteria which may establish a diagnosis of NTM lung infection. These criteria have not been validated in organ transplant recipients.

[b]Criteria for NTM prophylaxis and treatment regimens have not been systematically studied in organ transplant recipients. Lung transplant candidates colonized with MAC may develop MAC infection following transplant and should receive multidrug therapy prior to lung transplantation. Lung transplant candidates colonized by rapidly growing mycobacteria (RGM; *M. chelonae*, *M. abscessus* or *M. fortuitum*) should receive AZ prophylaxis (1200 mg PO/week) post-transplant to prevent infection.

[c]RGM should be identified to the species level due to differences in treatment recommendations and isolates should undergo susceptibility testing. Consider surgical debridement for localized non-pulmonary disease such as skin infection and remove catheters when infection is catheter-related.

[d]More than one agent is advised for initiation of therapy due to potential for development of antimicrobial resistance. For severe disease, treatment with three or more agents may be necessary. AZ is favored over CLARI and rifabutin favored over RIF due to fewer drug interactions with immunosuppressive medications such as cyclosporine and tacrolimus. Consider concomitant reduction in immunosuppression. Treat pulmonary disease until sputum cultures are negative over a 12-month period. Treat skin and soft tissue infections for 3–6 months, depending on severity of infection.

[e]Adjust doses for renal function as necessary.

[f]RIF has major interaction with calcineurin-inhibitors.

References: [1] *Am J Transplantation* 2009; **9**(s4): S63; [2] *Am J Respir Crit Care Med* 2007; **175**(4):367; [3] *Clin Infect Dis* 2004; **38**: 1428; [4] *Clin Infect Dis* 2001; **33**: 1433. [5] *Antimicrob Agents Chemother* 2008; **52**: 4184.

29 *Pneumocystis jiroveci* Pneumonia: Prophylaxis and Therapy

Nicolas J. Mueller

	Suggested regimens		Comments
	Primary	Alternative	
Prophylaxis			
	TMP-SMX, SS or DS[a], once/day *or* TMP-SMX DS three times/week (studied for PCP only, see comments)	Dapsone 50–100 mg/day *or* Aerosolized pentamidine 300 mg q4wk *or* Atovaquone 1500 mg/day	Duration: 6–12 months post-transplant, lifelong for lung transplants (some centers may give more prolonged for some transplants). Consider prophylaxis during and after treatment of acute rejection (duration 6 weeks)
			TMP-SMX has added benefit: *Toxoplasma gondii*, *Nocardia*, are mostly prevented as are some GI, UTI and respiratory tract infections.
			Dapsone: check G6PD deficiency in risk population
Therapy			
Outpatient treatment, able to take PO meds, *PaO₂* > 70 mmHg (>10 kPa)	TMP-SMX DS 2 Tbs PO q8h × 14–21 days *or* Dapsone 100 mg PO q24h + trimethoprim 5 mg/kg TID × 14–21 days	Primaquine 15–30 mg PO q24h + clindamycin 600 mg PO q8h × 14–21 days *or* Atovaquone suspension with food 750 mg PO BID × 14–21 days	Duration in non-AIDS patient not well studied, 14 days only with optimal clinical course and reduction of immune suppression Secondary prophylaxis recommended
Hospitalized patient, *PaO₂* < 70 mmHg (<10 kPa)	TMP-SMX 15 mg/kg/day of TMP component IV divided in three doses + prednisone (see comments) × 21 days	Primaquine 15–30 mg PO q24h + clindamycin 600 mg IV q8h × 21 days *or* Pentamidine 4 mg/kg/day × 21 days + prednisone (see comments)	Based on data from HIV patients: consider concomitant use of corticosteroids if *PaO₂* <70 mmHg: prednisone (start **before** TMP-SMX) 40 mg PO BID for 5 days, then 40 mg PO q24h for 5 days, then 20 mg PO q24h for 11 days)
			Less evidence of efficacy with alternative therapy
			Secondary prophylaxis recommended

AIDS, acquired immune deficiency syndrome; BID, twice daily; G6PD, glucose-6-phosphate dehydrogenase; GI, gastrointestinal; HIV, human immunodeficiency virus; IV, intravenous; PCP, *P. jiroveci* pneumonia; PO, by mouth; SMX, sulfamethoxazole; Tbs, tablets; TID, three times daily; TMP, trimethoprim; UTI, urinary tract infection
[a]DS, double strength: TMP, 160 mg/SMX, 800 mg; SS, single strength: TMP 80 mg/SMX 400 mg.

The AST Handbook of Transplant Infections, 1st edition. Edited by D. Kumar & A. Humar. © 2011 Blackwell Publishing Ltd.

30 Suggested Therapy of *Clostridium difficile* Colitis After Transplantation

Aneesh K. Mehta

Syndrome	Suggested treatment	Alternative	Comment
C. difficile colitis – mild to moderate	Metronidazole 500 mg PO TID × 14 days	Vancomycin 125–250 mg PO QID × 14 days	Diagnosis based on toxin A & B EIA or cytotoxicity assay/toxigenic culture or *C. difficile* PCR Rule out other pathogens (e.g. CMV, enteric pathogens) If testing negative, consider endoscopy and CT scan
C. difficile colitis – severe/toxic megacolon	Vancomycin 250 mg PO/NG QID *and* Metronidazole 500 mg IV TID	Consider vancomycin enema if unable to take PO/NG Consider adjunctive therapy with nitazoxanide (500 mg PO/NG BID) or rifaximin (400 mg PO/NG BID)	Decrease immunosuppression Surgical consultation; may need colectomy Consider IVIg (e.g. 500 mg/kg daily × 3 days)
Relapsing *C. difficile*	Vancomycin PO – may need prolonged therapy (e.g. 250 mg PO QID × 3–4 weeks) or tapering (see comments)	–	Consider discontinuation of prophylactic antibiotics (e.g. TMP/SMX) Decrease immunosuppression Tapering vancomycin course: 250 mg PO QID × 2 weeks 125 mg PO QID × 2 weeks 125 mg PO BID × 4 weeks

CMV, cytomegalovirus; CT, computed tomography; EIA, enzyme immunoassay; IV, intravenous; IVIg, intravenous immunoglobulin; NG, nasogastric tube; PCR, polymerase chain reaction ; PO, by mouth; QID, four times a day; SMX, sulfamethoxazole; TID, three times a day; TMP, trimethoprim.

The AST Handbook of Transplant Infections, 1st edition. Edited by D. Kumar & A. Humar. © 2011 Blackwell Publishing Ltd.

31 Diagnosis and Treatment of Multidrug-Resistant Bacteria

Emily A. Blumberg

Organism	Diagnosis	Treatment (*Adjust based on individual susceptibility testing*)[a–i]
Methicillin-resistant *Staphylococcus aureus* (MRSA)	Oxacillin MIC ≥4 μg/mL or methicillin MIC ≥16 μg/mL or disc diffusion with cefoxitin 30 μg disc zone size ≤19 mm Detection of *mec A* gene by molecular methods Vancomycin MIC ≤2 μg/mL	Vancomycin IV maintaining trough levels >10 μg/mL Some experts suggest maintaining trough >15 g/mL if MIC >1 μg/mL or if patient has complicated infection (e.g. bacteremia, endocarditis, pneumonia, meningitis) If vancomycin MIC ≥2 μg/mL, consider alternative therapy (assuming organism is susceptible): • Daptomycin (bacteremia, skin and soft tissue infections, endocarditis) • Linezolid (skin and soft tissue infections, pneumonia) • Quinupristin-dalfopristin (skin and soft tissue infections) • TMP-SMX (skin and soft tissue infections, osteomyelitis, pneumonia) • Clindamycin (skin and soft tissue infection, pneumonia, osteomyelitis) • Tigecycline (skin and soft tissue infections, peritonitis)[j]
Vancomycin-intermediate *Staphylococcus aureus* (VISA), heteroresistant VISA (hVISA)	Vancomycin MIC 4–8 μg/mL hVISA may have small subpopulations with higher MICs on vancomycin screen agar plates or disc diffusion methods	Avoid use of vancomycin Consider alternatives listed above if susceptible Infectious diseases consultation
Vancomycin-resistant *Staphylococcus aureus*	Vancomycin MIC ≥16 μg/mL	Avoid use of vancomycin Consider alternatives listed above if susceptible Infectious diseases consultation

(Continued)

The AST Handbook of Transplant Infections, 1st edition. Edited by D. Kumar & A. Humar. © 2011 Blackwell Publishing Ltd.

(Continued)

Organism	Diagnosis	Treatment (*Adjust based on individual susceptibility testing*)[a–i]
Vancomycin-resistant *Enterococci* (VRE)	Vancomycin MIC $\geqslant$ 32 μg/mL Screen isolates with MIC $\geqslant$ 8 μg/mL with PCR	Ampicillin is drug of choice for susceptible isolates For ampicillin-resistant isolates, consider alternative therapy, if susceptible: • Linezolid (bacteriostatic so may not be preferred for endovascular infection) • Daptomycin • Tigecycline (caution advised with bacteremia, UTI or high density infections)[j] • Quinupristin-dalfopristin (*Enterococcus faecium* only) • Tetracyclines (non-serious infections) • Fosfomycin (uncomplicated UTIs) • Nitrofurantoin (uncomplicated UTIs)
Multidrug-resistant *Enterobacteriaceae*	Extended spectrum beta-lactamase (ESBL) producers: • Double disk diffusion assay • Broth dilution with/without beta-lactamase inhibitor • ESBL E-test strip Carbapenemase producers: • Disk diffusion using ertapenem or meropenem • Microbroth dilution with ertapenem, meropenem, or imipenem	Carbapenems when susceptible Tigecycline (caution advised with bacteremia, UTI or high density infections)[j] Colistin (IV) Fosfomycin (uncomplicated UTIs)
Multidrug-resistant *Acinetobacter baumanii*	Individual carbapenem testing Tests vary for each antimicrobial	Carbapenems (except ertapenem) Ampicillin-sulbactam (note that amoxicillin-clavulanate is not an acceptable alternative) Tigecycline (caution advised with bacteremia, UTI or high density infections)[j] Colistin (IV) with/without carbapenem Fosfomycin (uncomplicated UTIs)
Multidrug-resistant *Pseudomonas aeruginosa*	MacConkey agar with cetirimide E-test or standardized disk diffusion	Consider initial therapy with combination of active beta-lactam and aminoglycoside or quinolone: • High-dose or continuous therapy may be warranted • Use of aerosolized aminoglycoside or colistin may be considered adjunctive for airway infections in lung transplant recipients Colistin for beta-lactam and aminoglycoside-resistant infection

Organism	Diagnosis	Treatment (*Adjust based on individual susceptibility testing*)[a–i]
Multidrug-resistant *Burkholderia cepacia*	OFPBL or *Pseudomonas cepacia* (PC) agar *Burkholderia cepacia* selective agar (BCSA)	TMP-SMX (high dose)
Multidrug-resistant *Stenotrophomonas maltophilia*	MacConkey agar	TMP-SMX (high dose) (drug of choice)
	VIA agar	Ceftazidime
	DNAse confirmatory media	Fluoroquinolones
	Biochemical molecular identification	Doxycycline (check susceptibility first)[j]
	E-test or standardized disk diffusion	
Multidrug-resistant *Achromobacter xylosoxidans*	E-test Standardized disk diffusion	Infectious diseases consultation

IV, intravenous; MIC, minimal inhibitory concentration; OFPBL, oxidation-fermentation polymyxin-bacitracin-lactose; PCR, polymerase chain reaction; TMP-SMX, trimethoprim-sulfamethoxazole; UTIs, urinary tract infections; VIA, vancomycin, imipenem, and amphotericin B.

[a]Infectious diseases consultation is recommended for all transplant recipients or candidates with multidrug-resistant bacterial infections.

[b]Multidrug-resistant bacteria should be suspected in patients with prolonged hospital stays (especially in ICU settings and burn units), exposure to broad-spectrum antibiotics, prior colonization with organism, proximity to other patients with resistant bacteria, and indwelling foreign objects (including intravascular devices).

[c]Close communication with the microbiology laboratory is essential to prompt identification of these organisms.

[d]All empirical antibiotic choices should be confirmed by specific antimicrobial susceptibility testing.

[e]Treatment should include removal of removable foci of infection (including intravascular devices, other foreign bodies) and debridement/drainage of wounds and affected tissue, where appropriate.

[f]Duration of treatment will vary with the organism and site but clinicians should treat using the shortest medically appropriate course of therapy.

[g]Patients should be closely monitored for signs of persistent infection as organisms may develop additional resistance on therapy.

[h]Contact isolation for patients with documented infection or colonization with these organisms.

[i]The risks of post-transplant complications should be considered in all transplant candidates who are colonized with multidrug-resistant bacteria and a modified perioperative antibacterial prophylaxis strategy should be considered.

[j]There was an FDA-warning in 2010 about the potential for increased mortality with tigecycline in severe infections.

References: [1] *Am J Transplantation* 2009; **9**(s4): S41; [2] *Am J Transplantation* 2009; **9**(s4): S50; [3] *Am J Transplantation* 2009; **9**(s4): S27.

32 Management of Selected Parasitic Infections After Transplant

Sanjay Mehta & Robert Huang

Pathogen	Treatment [1]	Alternatives
Protozoa		
Babesiosis (*Babesia* sp.)	Atovaquone 750 mg PO BID + azithromycin 500 mg PO daily × 7–10 days. Patients may be at risk for persistent/relapsing disease; requires prolonged treatment [2]	Clindamycin 600 mg PO/IV TID + quinine 650 mg PO TID
Balantidiasis (*Balantidium coli*)	Tetracycline 500 mg PO QID × 10 days *and/or* Metronidazole 750–1000 mg PO TID × 10 days	–
Cryptosporidiosis (*Cryptosporidium parvum* or *C. muris*)	Reduce immunosuppression Nitazoxanide 500 mg PO BID × 14 days	Azithromycin 600 mg PO daily + paromomycin 1 g PO BID
Cyclosporiasis (*Cyclospora* sp.)	TMP-SMX one tablet DS PO QID × 10 days then three times/wk	Ciprofloxacin 500 mg PO BID × 7 days then 500 mg three times/wk × 2 weeks
Amebiasis (*Entamoeba histolytica*)		
Intestinal	Metronidazole[a] 750 mg PO TID × 10 days followed by therapy for intestinal colonization	Tinidazole 2 g PO daily × 3 days
Extraintestinal	Metronidazole 750 mg PO TID × 10 days (or tinidazole) followed by therapy for intestinal colonization	Chloroquine 600 mg PO QD × 2 days then 300 mg PO BID for 20 days
Colonization	Paromomycin 25–35 mg/kg/day PO TID × 7 days	Iodoquinol 650 mg PO TID × 20 days
Giardiasis (*Giardia lamblia*)	Metronidazole 500 mg PO TID × 5 days *or* Tinidazole 2 g PO once	Nitazoxanide 500 mg PO BID × 3 days
Isosporiasis (*Isospora belli*)	TMP-SMX one tablet DS PO TID × 10 days followed by BID × 2–4 weeks	Ciprofloxacin 500 mg PO BID × 7 days *or* Pyrimethamine 50–75 mg PO daily + folinic acid 10 mg PO daily × 2 weeks

(Continued)

The AST Handbook of Transplant Infections, 1st edition. Edited by D. Kumar & A. Humar. © 2011 Blackwell Publishing Ltd.

Pathogen	Treatment [1]	Alternatives
Microsporidiosis		
CNS or disseminated	Albendazole 400 mg PO BID × 4 weeks For ocular disease, add fumagillin eye drops	
Intestinal	Albendazole 400 mg PO BID × 4 weeks	Fumagillin 20 mg PO TID (for *Enterocytozoon bieneusi* only)
Malaria (*Plasmodium falciparum or P. malariae*)		
Non-severe disease	*Chloroquine-sensitive*[b]: chloroquine 1 g salt (600 mg base) PO once then 0.5 g in 6 hours, then 0.5 g daily × 2 days. *Chloroquine-resistant*: atovaquone/proguanil 1 g/400 mg PO daily × 3 days	Chloroquine resistant: quinine sulfate 650 mg PO TID + doxycyline 100 mg PO BID × 7 days
Severe or cerebral malaria (*P. falciparum*)	Quinidine gluconate[b] 10 mg/kg IV over 1 hour infusion then 0.02 mg/kg/minute by constant infusion until parasite density < 1%, then switch to PO quinine sulfate	
Malaria (*P. vivax or P. ovale*)	Chloroquine-sensitive: chloroquine 1 g PO (600 mg base) once then 0.5 g in 6 hours, then 0.5 g QD × 2 days *and* Primaquine 30 mg base PO daily × 14 days to treat hepatic stage (check for G6PD deficiency prior to administration)	If chloroquine-RESISTANT: Quinine sulfate 650 mg PO TID + doxycycline 100 mg PO BID × 7 days + primaquine × 14 days
Toxoplasma gondii (also see SOT prophylaxis Table 40) disseminated/CNS acute encephalitis	Pyrimethamine 200 mg PO load then 50–75 mg PO daily + folinic acid 10–25 mg daily + sulfadiazine PO 1–1.5 g QID × 4–6 weeks, then suppressive therapy *or* TMP-SMX 5 mg/kg of TMP component BID × 30 days, then suppressive therapy	If sulfa allergic the following may be substituted: Clindamycin 600 mg PO/IV QID *or* Atovaquone 750 mg PO QID
Toxoplasma – suppression after treatment of acute infection	Pyrimethamine 25–50 mg PO daily + folinic acid 10–25 mg PO daily + sulfadiazine PO 2–4 g daily (in four divided doses)	TMP-SMX one tablet DS PO daily If sulfa allergic: Clindamycin 600 mg PO TID + pyrimethamine *or* Atovaquone 750 mg TID–QID

(Continued)

(*Continued*)

Pathogen	Treatment [1]	Alternatives
Chagas disease (*Trypanosoma cruzi*)	Nifurtimox 8–10 mg/kg PO daily divided in four doses × 90–120 days (call CDC for drug 1-404-639-2888) For recipients of organs other than hearts from seropositive donors consider either: benznidazole × 4–8 weeks [3] or pre-emptive therapy upon detection of parasitemia with benznidazole × 8 weeks For seropositive recipients: benznidazole × 4–8 weeks or pre-emptive therapy upon detection of parasitemia with benznidazole × 8 weeks	Benznidazole 5–7 mg/kg/day PO divided BID × 60 days Do not recommend acceptance of heart of donor seropositive for Chagas disease for transplantation
Helminths		
Schistosoma – *S. hematobium* (urinary), *S. intercalatum*, *S. japonicum*, *S. mansoni*, *S. mekongi*	Praziquantel 20 mg/kg PO BID × 1 day (TID for *S. japonicum* or *mekongi*) Check affected site for ova 1 month after treatment and retreat if still positive	Oxamniquine for *S. mansoni*
Strongyloidiasis (*Strongyloides stercoralis*)	Ivermectin 200 µg/kg/day × 2 days (uncomplicated intestinal disease) or × 7 days for disseminated disease	Albendazole 400 mg PO BID (same durations as ivermectin)
Neurocysticercosis (*Taenia solium*) – parenchymal neuro-cysticercosis or degenerating cyst	Albendazole: *<60 kg* – 400 mg PO BID with meals *<60 kg* – 15/mg/kg/day in two divided doses (max. 800 mg/day) + dexamethasone 0.1 mg/kg per day + anti-seizure medication[c] × 30 days No treatment for dead calcified cyst	Praziquantel 100 mg/kg/day in three divided doses then 50 mg/kg/day in three divided doses + dexamethasone 0.1 mg/kg/day + anti-seizure medication × 30 days

BID, twice daily; CSF, cerebrospinal fluid; CNS, central nervous system; DS, double strength; G6PD, glucose-6-phosphate dehydrogenase; IV, intravenous; PO, by mouth; QD, once a day; QID, four times a day; SOT, solid organ transplant; TID, three times daily; TMP-SMX, trimethoprim-sulfamethoxazole.

Leishmaniasis and helminths such as *Paragonimus*, *Fasciola*, *Clonorchis* are not covered. For these, refer to other sources or tropical disease experts.

[a]Metronidazole may increase levels of cyclosporine and tacrolimus; levels should be monitored. Metronidazole may decrease levels of mycophenolic acid.

[b]Chloroquine and mefloquine + tacrolimus may increase QT intervals.

[c]Anti-seizure medications such as phenytoin and carbemazepine significantly decrease calcineurin inhibitor levels and levels should be monitored if these drugs are used.

References (in square brackets): [1] *Am J Transplantation* 2009; 9(s4):S234; [2] *Clin Infect Dis* 2008; 46(3): 370; [3] *Am J Transplantation* 2007; 7(3): 680.

PART III
Donor Issues

33 Infectious Disease Evaluation of the Potential Organ Donor

Staci A. Fischer

Routine screening of all donors

- Cytomegalovirus (CMV) immunoglobulin G (IgG)
- Epstein–Barr virus (EBV) IgG
- Human immunodeficiency virus (HIV) antibody
- Hepatitis C antibody (HCV)
- Hepatitis B (HBV): hepatitis B surface antigen (HbsAg), hepatitis B core antibody (anti-Hbc)
- Syphilis (e.g. rapid plasma reagin)
- Human T-cell lymphotrophic virus (HTLV)-I/II antibody (previously required but no longer routinely done in US)

In deceased donors
- Blood cultures
- Urine cultures
- Sputum or bronchoalveolar lavage cultures (especially if lungs utilized)

Optional donor testing

- Nucleic acid testing for HIV, hepatitis B and/or hepatitis C
- West Nile virus (WNV) nucleic acid testing (NAT)
- Herpes simplex virus (HSV) antibody
- *Toxoplasma* antibody (heart donors)
- *Trypanosoma cruzi* antibody in donors from endemic areas (e.g. Mexico, Central America, South America)
- *Coccidioides* antibody in donors from endemic areas (e.g. south-western US, Mexico, Central America, South America)
- *Histoplasma* antibody in donors from endemic areas (e.g. Ohio and Mississippi river valleys in US, other river valleys in North and Central America, Eastern and southern Europe, Africa and Australia)
- *Strongyloides* antibody in donors from endemic areas (e.g. Appalachian US, Central America, South America, sub-Saharan Africa, South-east Asia, eastern Europe)
- *Brucella* serology in donors from endemic areas (e.g. Middle East, Mediterranean basin, eastern Europe, Asia, Africa, Central and South America). Ingestion of unpasteurized milk or cheeses from endemic areas is a risk factor for infection
- Human herpes virus-8 (HHV-8) serology
- BK virus serology (kidney donors)

Additional considerations in the deceased donor

- Caution should be used when utilizing organs from deceased donors with encephalitis, meningitis, or flaccid paralysis of undetermined etiology, as viruses such as rabies, lymphocytic choriomeningitis virus (LCMV) and WNV have been transmitted from deceased donors in recent years.
- There is a theoretical risk of transmission of other more common viral infections (e.g. influenza) in patients with active infection at the time of donation. Nasopharyngeal swab testing with respiratory viral panels may be helpful to rule out infections such as influenza, adenovirus, and respiratory syncytial virus if there is clinical suspicion.
- Tuberculosis (TB) may be transmitted by latently infected organ donors.

The AST Handbook of Transplant Infections, 1st edition. Edited by D. Kumar & A. Humar. © 2011 Blackwell Publishing Ltd.

Clues to the presence of infection in the deceased organ donor

- History of homosexual male or intravenous drug use or sexual contact with the above: HIV, HBV, HCV
- History of incarceration: TB, HIV, HBV, HCV
- Cocaine snorting: HCV
- Rash: possible viral infection
- Stiff neck: meningitis
- Tattoos: HIV, HBV, HCV
- Track marks (suggestive of active intravenous drug usage): HIV, HBV, HCV
- Fever, mental status changes, or other signs of potential infection should be evaluated thoroughly in the potential organ donor. Informed consent of the recipient of any identified or potential infections should be obtained.

Screening of the potential living donor

- Thorough medical, social and geographic history to identify potential exposures to infections which can be transmitted.

- Serologic and other testing is indicated for the donor with a history of residence or prolonged stay in an endemic area for certain infections (see 'Optional donor testing' above).
- Screening for latent tuberculosis with purified protein derivative (PPD) testing or interferon-gamma release assays should be done in all donors. In those from highly endemic areas such as Africa, Asia and Central and South America, a two-stage PPD (testing 4 weeks apart) may be indicated.

Resources

[1] *Am J Transplantation* 2009; 9(s4): S7 – updated guidelines on screening donors and recipients
[2] *Clin Microbiol Rev* 2008; 21: 60–96.
[3] http://optn.transplant.hrsa.gov/PoliciesandBylaws2/policies/pdfs/policy_16.pdf – current United Network for Organ Sharing (UNOS) policies concerning donor-transmitted infection prevention.
[4] www.cdc.gov/travel/yellowbook/2010 – updated information on travel-related infections with details on areas of endemicity for the pathogens noted above.

34 Infectious Disease Evaluation of the Potential Hematopoietic Stem Cell Transplant Donor

Staci A. Fischer

Routine screening of all donors

- Cytomegalovirus (CMV) immunoglobulin G (IgG)
- Epstein–Barr virus (EBV) IgG
- Human immunodeficiency virus (HIV) antibody, nucleic acid testing (NAT)
- Hepatitis C: antibody, NAT
- Hepatitis B: hepatitis B surface antigen (HbsAg), hepatitis B core antibody (anti-Hbc)
- Herpes simplex virus (HSV) IgG
- Syphilis screening (e.g. rapid plasma reagin)

Optional donor testing

- Hepatitis B NAT
- Human T-cell lymphotrophic virus (HTLV)-I/II antibodies
- West Nile virus (WNV) NAT
- *Toxoplasma* antibody
- *Trypanosoma cruzi* antibody in donors from endemic areas (e.g. Mexico, Central America, South America)
- *Strongyloides* antibody in donors from endemic areas (e.g. Appalachian US, Central America, South America, sub-Saharan Africa, Southeast Asia, eastern Europe)
- *Leishmania* antibody or polymerase chain reaction (PCR) in donors with travel to or residence in an endemic area (e.g. Iraq, central and South America, Indian subcontinent, Middle East, East Africa)
- Thin and thick malaria preparations in donors from endemic areas (e.g. central and South America, Haiti, Dominican Republic, Africa, Asia, Eastern Europe)
- *Babesia* serology in donors from endemic areas (e.g. New England, upper Midwest in the US)
- *Rickettsia* serology and/or PCR in donors from endemic areas (see www.cdc.gov)
- *Coxiella burnetii* serology in paitents with extensive exposure to cattle, sheep and goats (Q fever)

Comments

- Serologic testing of HSCT donors should be done within 30 days of donation, with repeat screening for possible acute infection performed within a week prior to donation.
- There is no known risk of tuberculosis transmission from donors with untreated latent TB infection, so that TB testing is not necessary.
- It is critical that a careful travel history be performed to identify potential donor-transmitted pathogens (see 'Optional donor testing' above).
- People with a history of deferral for blood donation, as well as those with prior corneal or dura mater transplantation, human pituitary-derived growth hormone administration, or 3–6 months or longer residence in the UK between 1980 and 1996 should be investigated further.

Resources

[1] *MMWR* 2000; 49(RR10): 1–128 – comprehensive guidelines for prevention of infection in HSCT.

The AST Handbook of Transplant Infections, 1st edition. Edited by D. Kumar & A. Humar. © 2011 Blackwell Publishing Ltd.

[2] http://www.fda.gov/BiologicsBloodVaccines/Safety Availability/TissueSafety/ucm095440.htm – *Testing HCT/P Donors for Relevant Communicable Disease Agents and Diseases* – updated guidelines for testing blood and HSCT donors for infectious including information on specific FDA-approved assays

[3] www.aabb.org/Content/Blood_Donor_History_ Questionnaires/HPC-Donor_History_Questionnaire – updated questionnaire for potential blood and HSCT donors, including algorithms for inclusion/exclusion criteria based on results of infection testing

[4] www.advanceweb.com/MLP – blood donor screening process and infectious disease testing using molecular methods. ADVANCE for Medical Laboratory Professionals 2007.

[5] www.cdc.gov/travel/yellowbook/2010 – updated information on travel-related infections with details on areas of endemicity for the pathogens noted above

35 Donor-derived Infections

Michael G. Ison

35.1 Potential infections that may be transmitted from donor to recipient [1,2]

- Infection of central nervous system
  - Viral encephalitis (e.g. JC, West Nile virus, rabies, HSV)
  - Parasitic encephalitis
  - Fungal encephalitis
  - Meningitis or other bacterial CNS infection
- Viral hepatitis (A, B, C, or E)
- West Nile virus infection
- Creutzfeldt–Jakob disease
- Infection with HIV
- Active viremia: herpes, acute EBV (mononucleosis)
- HTLV-I/II
- Parasitic infections (e.g. *Trypanosoma cruzi*, *Leishmania*, *Strongyloides*, *Toxoplasma*)
- Active tuberculosis
- SARS
- Pneumonia
- Bacterial or fungal sepsis (e.g. candidemia)
- Syphilis
- Endemic mycoses

CNS, central nervous system; EBV, Epstein–Barr virus; HIV, human immunodeficiency virus; HSV, herpes simplex virus; HTLV, human T-cell lymphotrophic virus; SARS, severe acute respiratory syndrome.

Notes:

1. Expected transmissions are those, such as EBV, cytomegalovirus, hepatitis B virus (HBV), hepatitis C virus (HCV), and toxoplasmosis, in which routine screening tests detect the latent infection of the donor. These expected infections are transmitted regularly by transplanted organs and their impact is mitigated through monitoring recipients for early infection or the use of universal prophylaxis.
2. Unexpected transmissions occur from a pathogen that was either unrecognized or not screened for in the donor, e.g. Chagas, HIV, HCV, lymphocytic choriomeningitis virus, *Mycobacterium tuberculosis*, rabies, and West Nile virus. Many of the unexpected transmissions have resulted in clinically significant morbidity and mortality.

References (in square brackets): [1] *Adv Chronic Kidney Dis* 2009;16:234; [2] American Transplant Congress (*ATC*) 2008 abst LB-02.

35.2 Management of specific donor scenarios

Scenario	Actions	Comments
Bacteremia in donor	Assess pathogen and susceptibility pattern If probable infection (coagulase-negative *Staphylococcus* may be contaminant – must contextualize with number of positive cultures and clinical picture of donor), would provide 2 weeks of active therapy, based on susceptibility patterns, in each recipient	Catastrophic outcomes, including mycotic aneurysms of the anastomosis site, graft loss, or sepsis can occur if bacteremia is not treated with an active antimicrobial [1, 4]
Bacterial meningitis in donor	Patients with culture-proven bacterial meningitis can be used safely as an organ donor if: • donor was appropriately treated for 24-48 hours with an antimicrobial active against the isolated organism • donor had an appropriate clinical response to therapy (improvement in temperature) • recipient receives a complete treatment course (typically 14 days) directed against the cultured pathogen	Culture-negative patients with a clinical picture consistent with bacterial meningitis have resulted in disease transmission, including a case of lymphoma [1, 4] Patient and graft survival similar in meningitis donors and non-infected donors [5]
Encephalitis	In general, donors with encephalitis should not be used unless there is a culture-positive bacterial cause If a donor with encephalitis is considered, the local transplant infectious diseases expert should be consulted before acceptance of the donor	Transmission of *Balamuthia*, LCMV, rabies, and West Nile virus are a few examples of infections transmitted from patients who died of non-bacterial encephalitis [1, 4] There are several reports of people with *Naegleria fowleri* encephalitis being successfully used as donors. If such donors are used, consent of the recipient must be obtained pre-transplant and infectious diseases expert should be consulted as early as possible [6]
Donor with pneumonia	Presence of pneumonia is typically a contraindication to lung transplantation; lungs that have completed a course of active antibacterial therapy may considered on a case-by-case basis If bacterial colonization is recognized on procurement cultures, pathogen-directed treatment should be considered for lung transplant recipients while treatment of other recipients is typically unnecessary unless there is evidence of bacteremia or fungemia	Fungal pneumonia is a contraindication to transplantation; *Candida* species typically do not cause pneumonia and positive respiratory cultures typically represent upper airway colonization
Donor with influenza	Influenza is typically an infection limited to the respiratory tract except in the setting of severe influenza or novel influenza virus infections. As such, risk is highest among lung recipients. Most recommend not using the lungs from donors with confirmed influenza (seasonal or pandemic) unless they have completed a standard course of therapy. Use of other organs could be considered on a case-by-case basis	There have been at least two confirmed cases of donor-derived influenza transmission involving infected lungs If virus is transmitted from an organ other than the lung, an atypical presentation may be expected – including fever and local symptoms; respiratory symptoms may be absent. Collection of alternative samples, including blood, urine, and stool, should be considered

(Continued)

Scenario	Actions	Comments
	All recipients of organs from a donor with confirmed influenza should receive empiric treatment (not prophylaxis) with an active antiviral for at least 5 days post-transplant	
Donor with UTI	Presence of a UTI does not rule out a donor; donors with pyelonephritis may be at higher risk of transmitting infection and the condition should be discussed with the accepting nephrologist	–
	Typically, kidney transplant recipients would need to receive a 3–7 day course of antibiotics active against the uropathogen; treatment of other recipients is likely unnecessary unless there is evidence of bacteremia or fungemia	
Donor with positive syphilis screen	People with positive syphilis serology can safely be used as donors. Confirmatory testing with *Treponema*-specific test (such as FTA-ABS) should be done to r/o a false-positive screening test	If the recipient is penicillin allergic, consult local infectious diseases expert for appropriate therapy
	Prior history of treated STDs, including syphilis, in the donor should be obtained. Irrespective of donor STD history, all recipients of donors with confirmed positive syphilis serology should receive appropriate therapy for syphilis of unclear duration – typically penicillin G 2.4 million units IM weekly for 3 weeks	
Donor with Chagas	Any donor with a positive Chagas serology should be confirmed by secondary testing (typically a RIPA) because of poor specificity of the test	In the US, medication for Chagas is available only through CDC (http://www.cdc.gov/chagas/)
	Any recipient of organs from a donor confirmed to be infected with Chagas by serology should be monitored for evidence of Chagas replication and treated with the first evidence of replication	In the US, the CDC should be contacted as soon as Chagas is recognized in the donor
Donor with *Strongyloides*	Although *Strongyloides* serology is rarely obtained on donors, if it is positive or if an O&P examination of stool reveals *Strongyloides*, the recipient should receive two doses of ivermectin 0.2 mg/kg 1 week between doses	–
Donor with tuberculosis [7]	Active tuberculosis is a contraindication to transplantation	–
	Management of donors with latent TB or granulomatous disease is more complicated (see Chapter 39)	

(*Continued*)

(Continued)

Donor with positive HTLV serology [3]	Any positive donor HTLV-1/2 serology needs to have confirmation because of poor specificity. If the donor is confirmed to be HTLV-1-infected, the recipient should have baseline HTLV serology drawn (if not already done) Optimal monitoring and management protocols have not been established; would consult local infectious diseases expert	Current serologic tests lack significant specificity and cannot differentiate between HTLV-1, which may be associated with disease in humans, and HTLV-2, which may not be associated with clinical disease
Donor with other documented infections	Discuss the donor and his/her specific issues with the OPO medical director and the accepting clinician [2]	–

FT-ABS, fluorescent treponemal antibody absorbed; HTLV, human T-cell lymphotrophic virus ; IM, intramuscular; LCMV, lymphocytic choriomeningitis virus; O&P, ova and parasite; OPO, organ procurement organization; RIPA, radioimmune precipitation assay; STD, sexually transmitted disease.

In all cases of donor infection, consult with your local transplant infectious diseases or infectious diseases expert. Always obtain an infectious diseases consult on the recipient immediately post-transplant if there is any concern for a donor-derived infection.

References (in square brackets): [1] *Adv Chronic Kidney Dis* 2009; 16: 234; [2] *OPTN Policy 4*; [3] *Am J Transplantation* 2010; 10(2): 207; [4] *ATC* 2008 abst LB-02; [5] *Transplantation* 2001; 72: 1108; [6] *Am J Transplantation* 2008; 8: 1334; [7] *Clin Infect Dis* 2009; 48: 1276.

36 Estimates of Window Period[a] Length for Serology and Nucleic Acid Testing

Atul Humar

Pathogen	Standard serology	Nucleic acid testing
Human immunodeficiency virus (HIV)	17–22 days	5–6 days
Hepatitis C virus (HCV)	~ 70 days	3–5 days
Hepatitis B virus (HBV)	35–44 days	20–22 days

[a]Window period = time from onset of infection to the detection of infection by a specific testing method.

HIV, HCV and HBV NAT data are listed for the most sensitive NAT currently used in blood donor screening (Gen Probe TMA for HIV and HCV, and Roche Cobas MPX for HBV on individual donation); the window period will be longer if less sensitive NAT is used for donor screening.

Reference: *Am J Transplantation* 2010; 10(4): 889.

The AST Handbook of Transplant Infections, 1st edition. Edited by D. Kumar & A. Humar. © 2011 Blackwell Publishing Ltd.

37 Estimates of Residual Risk of HIV or HCV when using Selected Increased Risk Donor Categories[a]

Atul Humar

Type of behaviour	Standard serology residual risk		Nucleic acid testing residual risk	
	HIV risk	HCV risk	HIV risk	HCV risk
Intravenous drug use	0.5–2.1/1000	14–65/1000	0.2–0.6/1000	1.4–6.5/1000
Prison inmate	0.1–0.2/1000	0.8–2.1/1000	0.04–0.08/1000	0.08–0.2/1000
Men who have sex with men	0.1–4.8/1000	1.3/1000	0.04–1.5/1000	0.1/1000
Commercial sex trade worker	9.8–11.4/1000	Limited data	3.1–3.6/1000	Limited data

HCV, hepatitis C virus; HIV, human immunodeficiency virus.

[a]These are only estimates. These data are derived from various incidence studies in the non-organ donor population. There are very few specific data about residual risk in organ donors. Risk assumes that the high-risk behaviour is being carried out right until the point of organ donation. Risk for hepatitis B virus (HBV) also exists. Fewer data are available about incident HBV infection than about HIV or HCV in various risk groups.

References: [1] *Am J Transplantation* 2010; 10(4): 889; [2] *Am J Transplantation* 2007; 7(6): 1515.

38 Management of Recipients of Hepatitis B Core Antibody-Positive Donor Organ

Karen E. Doucette

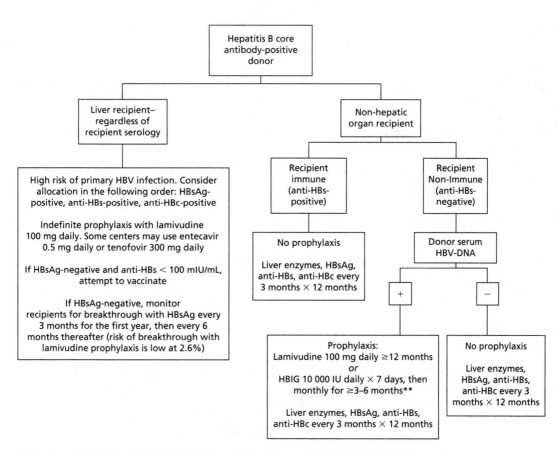

anti-HBs, hepatitis B surface antibody; HBsAg, hepatitis B surface antigen; HBV, hepatitis B virus.

References: [1] *J Hepatol* 2010; 52(2): 272; [2] *Am J Transplantation* 2001; 1: 185; [3] *Am J Transplantation* 2009; 9(s4): S116.

The AST Handbook of Transplant Infections, 1st edition. Edited by D. Kumar & A. Humar. © 2011 Blackwell Publishing Ltd.

39 Donor Tuberculosis Issues: Potential Scenarios and Management

Camille N. Kotton & Michele I. Morris

Type	Risk for transmission	Recommendation	
		Living donor	Deceased donor
Latent TB			
Donor has history of TB exposure or significant risk factors for TB but has not been tested	Variable	Test with TST or IGRA	Insufficient data on testing; monitor recipient clinically
Donor has history of latent TB and has been treated appropriately	Low	Monitor recipient clinically	Monitor recipient clinically
Donor has history of latent TB that was treated insufficiently or not treated or treatment details not clear *or* New diagnosis of latent TB (by TST or IGRA); no evidence of active TB	Moderate	Consider deferring transplant if possible until donor has taken some/all of prophylaxis and consider prophylaxis of recipient (recommend with lung)	Monitor recipient clinically; consider prophylaxis of recipient
Unexplained pulmonary apical fibrosis in donor without cavitation and without additional testing	Variable	Defer donation pending further evaluation	Consider in context of donor history/epidemiology. Consider bronchoscopy. If tests for TB are negative, accept as non-lung donor. Consider recipient prophylaxis
Active TB			
Donor has history of active TB: site remote from transplant (i.e. pulmonary in a kidney donor) – treated appropriately	Low to moderate	Monitor clinically; consider cultures of previous TB sites if possible; if TB was treated recently (< 2 years), consider recipient prophylaxis	Same as for living donor
Donor has history of active TB: site remote from transplant – inadequate treatment	Moderate to high	Defer live donors until adequately treated	Culture previous TB sites in the donor; recommend recipient prophylaxis
Donor has history of active TB: site same as transplant (i.e. renal TB in a kidney donor) – treated appropriately	Moderate	Verify treatment; give prophylaxis to recipient; cultures of previous TB site(s) if possible	Same as for living donor

(Continued)

The AST Handbook of Transplant Infections, 1st edition. Edited by D. Kumar & A. Humar. © 2011 Blackwell Publishing Ltd.

Type	Risk for transmission	Recommendation	
		Living donor	Deceased donor
Donor has history of active TB: site same as transplant – inadequate treatment	High	Defer live donors until adequately treated	Recommend rejecting donor; may consider in high-status/urgent recipients, and treat recipient for active TB with informed consent
Active TB in any organ at time of proposed donation	High	Reject; may re-evaluate after adequate treatment	Reject

IGRA, interferon-gamma release assays; TST, tuberculin skin test.

PART IV

Prevention of Infections after Transplantation

40 Suggested Prophylaxis Regimens in Organ Transplant Recipients

Nasia Safdar, Germana L.M. Silva & Jennifer Hsu

Pathogen/organ	Prophylactic regimens/comments
Cytomegalovirus (see Chapter 14 for more details)	
Heart, kidney, liver, pancreas	Valganciclovir 900 mg PO daily *or* ganciclovir 1 g PO TID for 3 months *or* valacyclovir 2 g PO QID (kidney only) *or* pre-emptive therapy
	Universal prophylaxis is preferred over pre-emptive therapy for D+/R–. Consider 6 months' prophylaxis for D+/R–
	Note: valganciclovir is not FDA-approved for liver transplantation, but many centers use it
Lung, heart–lung (D+/R–, R+)	Ganciclovir 5 mg/kg IV daily *or* valganciclovir 900 mg PO daily × 3–12 months
	Universal prophylaxis is preferred
	Some centers add CMVIg (e.g. 150 mg/kg within 72 hours and at 2, 4, 6, and 8 weeks post-transplant) in high-risk patients. A recent study showed that 12 months better than 3 months
Hepatitis B virus (see Chapter 22 for more details) – liver	HbsAg-positive recipients: indefinite nucleos(t)ide analogue therapy ± HBIg. Discontinuation of HBIg may be considered in patients with low/undetectable HBV DNA at transplant
	anti-HBc-positive recipients: indefinite nucleos(t)ide analogue therapy
HSV/VZV – all organs	Acyclovir 200 mg PO TID or 400–800 mg BID *or* valacyclovir 500 mg PO BID *or* famciclovir 250–500 mg PO BID × ≥ 1 month. Not necessary if receiving prophylaxis for CMV
Aspergillus sp. (Also see Chapters 11 and 25)	
Liver[a]	Lipid formulation of amphotericin B (3–5 mg/kg/day) *or* an echinocandin. Duration: initial hospital stay or for 4 weeks post-transplant.
	Risk factors: retransplantation, renal failure requiring renal replacement therapy, reoperation, transplant for fulminant hepatic failure
Lung[a]	Voriconazole 200 mg PO BID *or* inhaled amphotericin B 10–20 mg BID *or* inhaled ABLC 50 mg/day × 4 days followed by 50 mg/week *or* inhaled L-AmB 25 mg three times per week for the first 60 days after transplantation, 25 mg /week between 60 and 180 days, and 25 mg once every 2 weeks thereafter *or* itraconazole 200 mg PO BID. Duration is guided by airway inspection, surveillance respiratory cultures, and risk factors
	Risk factors include: *Aspergillus* colonization, CMV, rejection, airway ischemia
Heart[a]	Itraconazole 200 mg PO BID *or* voriconazole 200 mg PO BID for 50–150 days
	Risk factors: *Aspergillus* colonization, CMV disease, renal replacement therapy

(Continued)

The AST Handbook of Transplant Infections, 1st edition. Edited by D. Kumar & A. Humar. © 2011 Blackwell Publishing Ltd.

(Continued)

Pathogen/organ	Prophylactic regimens/comments
Candida sp.	
Liver	Fluconazole 200-400 mg IV/PO daily *or* echinocandin
	Risk factors: reoperation; retransplantation; renal failure; massive transfusion, biliary complications, *Candida* colonization.
	Duration: 4 weeks but adjust according to ongoing risk
	Observing liver transplant recipients with low risk for invasive fungal infection is safe. Use of fluconazole prophylaxis is associated with increased rate of non-*albicans Candida* infections
Small bowel	Fluconazole 200-400 mg IV/PO daily × 4 weeks but adjust according to ongoing risk; continue until anastomosis is healed and rejection is not present
	Consider use of echinocandin or L-AmB if risk factors for non-*albicans Candida* are present
Pancreas	Can consider fluconazole 200–400 g IV/PO daily for patients with risk factors including colonization, intra-abdominal abscess, vascular thrombosis, and pancreatitis
	Optimal duration: adjust according to risk factors
	Consider use of echinocandin or L-AmB if risk factors for non-*albicans Candida* are present
Kidney, heart, lung	No recommendation for *Candida* prophylaxis
Coccidioides immitis – all organs	If there is past history of *Coccidioides* infection or POSITIVE serologies, give fluconazole 200–400 mg IV/PO daily
	Same regimen for active infection/positive serologies in organ donor
	Duration: unknown, may be indefinite in some
Pneumocystis jiroveci – all organs	*First line*: TMP-SMX 1 SS tab PO daily or 1 DS tab PO three times/week[b]. Duration: for renal and liver, 6–12 months; for lung, lifelong; for heart, may depend on risk of toxoplasmosis
	Second line: dapsone 50–100 mg PO daily *or* atovaquone 1500 mg PO daily *or* aerosolized pentamidine 300 mg q3-4 weeks. Daily TMP-SMX regimens may be effective for prevention of other post-transplant infections, such as *Toxoplasma*, *Nocardia*, *Listeria*, common respiratory, urinary, and GI pathogens. Dapsone is contraindicated in G6PD deficiency
Toxoplasma gondii – heart (D+/R– or R+)	*First line*: TMP-SMX 1 SS tab PO daily or 1 DS tab PO three times/week. If D+/R– for *Toxoplasma*, can consider 1 DS tab PO daily, but preceding doses should be adequate. Optimal duration unknown; lifelong for D+/R–
	Second line: pyrimethamine and folinic acid.

ABLC, amphotericin B lipid complex; BID, twice daily; CMV, cytomegalovirus; D+/R–, donor positive/recipient negative; GI, gastrointestinal; anri-HBc, hepatitis B core antibody; HBV, hepatitis B virus; HSV, herpes simplex virus; Ig, immunoglobulin; L-AmB, liposomal amphotericin B; PO, by mouth; QD, once a day; QID, four times daily; R+, recipient positive; TID, three times daily; TMP-SMX, trimethoprim- sulfamethoxazole; VZV, varicella zoster virus.

[a]For all organs, target prophylaxis for high-risk patients.

[b]DS, double strength: TMP, 160 mg/SMX, 800 mg; SS, single strength: TMP 80 mg/SMX 400 mg.

References: [1] *Am J Transplantation* 2009; 9(s4): S78; [2] *Am J Transplantation* 2009; 9(s4): S116; [3] *Am J Transplantation* 2009; 9(s4): S108; [4] *Am J Transplantation* 2009; 9(s4): S104; [5] *Am J Transplantation* 2009; 9(s4): S180; [6] *Am J Transplantation* 2009; 9(s4): S173; [7] *Am J Transplantation* 2009; 9(s4): S199; [8] *Am J Transplantation* 2009; 9(s4): S227; [9] *Am J Transplantation* 2009; 9(s4): S234.

41 Antimicrobial Prophylaxis Regimen for Allogeneic Hematopoietic Stem Cell Transplant Recipients

Sherif Mossad

	Pre-engraftment (< 3 weeks)	Early post-engraftment (3 weeks–3 months) and late post-engraftment (>3 months)
Bacterial	Levofloxacin 500 mg PO or IV (due to mucositis) daily, or ciprofloxacin 500 mg PO BID Consider IVIg if IgG < 400 mg/dL	Amoxicillin 250 mg PO BID or azithromycin 250 mg PO daily (if allergic to penicillin) for ≥ 6 months; as long as immunosuppressive therapy is being administered Consider IVIg if IgG < 400 mg/dL
Fungal	Nystatin PO 500 000 units QID, or clotrimazole troches 10 mg PO TID, or amphotericin B suspension 500 mg PO QID, for oral mucosal prophylaxis Fluconazole 400 mg PO daily, or itraconazole solution 200 mg PO BID, or voriconazole 200 mg PO BID, or posaconazole 200 mg PO TID, or micafungin 50 mg IV QD, or 'low dose' amphotericin B[a] (0.2 mg/kg/day) for systemic prophylaxis	Itraconazole[b] solution 200 mg PO BID, or voriconazole 200 mg PO BID, or posaconazole[c] 200 mg PO TID, or micafungin 50 mg IV daily, or amphotericin B[a] 0.5 mg/kg IV every other day for ≥ 6 months, as long as immunosuppressive therapy is being administered Routine monitoring of azole drug levels is controversial, but should be considered in patients with breakthrough infections
Viral	Acyclovir 400 mg PO BID, or famciclovir 250 mg PO BID, or valacyclovir 500 mg PO BID, or 2 g PO QID (if used for CMV prophylaxis) Weekly surveillance CMV antigenemia or CMV PCR, and pre-emptive treatment with IV ganciclovir, or alternative agent	Continue acyclovir, famciclovir, or valacyclovir for 1 year, unless ganciclovir or valganciclovir are used for CMV pre-emptive treatment or universal prophylaxis For CMV seropositive donors or recipients: • Weekly surveillance CMV antigenemia or CMV PCR for ≥ 6 months, as long as immunosuppressive therapy is being administered, and pre-emptive treatment with IV ganciclovir, oral valganciclovir, or alternative agent (foscarnet or cidofovir) for at least 2 weeks; until surveillance test turns negative *or* • Universal prophylaxis with IV ganciclovir 5 mg/kg/day, or valganciclovir 900 mg PO daily for 3 months after transplant

(Continued)

The AST Handbook of Transplant Infections, 1st edition. Edited by D. Kumar & A. Humar. © 2011 Blackwell Publishing Ltd.

(Continued)

	Pre-engraftment (< 3 weeks)	Early post-engraftment (3 weeks–3 months) and late post-engraftment (>3 months)
Pneumocystis jiroveci	Early prophylaxis is controversial due to risk of delayed engraftment with TMP-SMX	TMP-SMX 160/800 mg PO daily, or pentamidine 300 mg inhaled monthly, or dapsone 100 mg PO daily, or atovaquone 1500 mg PO daily for ≥ 6 months, as long as immunosuppressive therapy is being administered

BID, twice daily; CMV, cytomegalovirus; D+/R–, donor positive/recipient negative; GI, gastrointestinal; IgG, immuno-globulin G; IVIg, intravenous immunoglobulin; PCR, polymerase chain reaction; PO, by mouth; QD, once a day; QID, four times daily; TID, three times daily; TMP-SMX, trimethoprim-sulfamethoxazole.

[a]Lipid formulations of amphotericin B may be substituted for conventional amphotericin B in patients with renal insufficiency.

[b]Itraconazole solution should be taken on an empty stomach, and is better absorbed than itraconazole tablets taken with acidic fluid such as orange juice or cola drink.

[c]Posaconazole should be taken with high-fat food or liquid nutritional supplement.

42 Antimicrobial Prophylaxis Regimen for Autologous Hematopoietic Stem Cell Transplant Recipients

Sherif Mossad

	Pre-engraftment (< 3 weeks)	Early post-engraftment (3 weeks–3 months) and late post-engraftment (> 3 months)
Bacterial	Levofloxacin 500 mg daily PO or IV (due to mucositis), or ciprofloxacin 500 mg BID Consider IVIg 400 mg/kg if IgG < 400 mg/dL	None
Fungal	Nystatin PO 500 000 units QID, or clotrimazole troches 10 mg PO TID, or amphotericin B suspension 500 mg PO QID, for oral mucosal prophylaxis Fluconazole 400 mg PO daily, or micafungin 50 mg IV daily, for systemic prophylaxis	Consider secondary prophylaxis for patients with previously confirmed invasive fungal infections
Viral	Acyclovir 400 mg PO BID, or famciclovir 250 mg PO BID, or valacyclovir 500 mg PO BID	Continue acyclovir, famciclovir, or valacyclovir for 1 year, unless ganciclovir or valganciclovir are used for CMV pre-emptive treatment or universal prophylaxis For CMV-seropositive patients who receive TBI, T-cell depleted grafts, or those who received alemtuzumab, fludarabine, or 2-CDA within 6 months prior to transplant, consider weekly surveillance CMV antigenemia or CMV PCR for ≥ 2 months, and pre-emptive treatment with IV ganciclovir, oral valganciclovir, or alternative agent (foscarnet or cidofovir) for at least 2 weeks, until surveillance test becomes negative
Pneumocystis jiroveci	Early prophylaxis is controversial due to risk of delayed engraftment with TMP-SMX	For patients with underlying leukemia, lymphoma, or myeloma who receive TBI, high-dose corticosteroids, T-cell-depleted grafts, or those who received alemtuzumab, fludarabine, or 2-CDA within 6 months prior to transplant, administer TMP-SMX 160/800 mg PO daily, or pentamidine 300 mg inhaled monthly, or dapsone 100 mg PO daily, or atovaquone 1500 mg PO daily for ≥ 6 months

BID, twice daily; CDA, chlorodeoxyadenosine; CMV, cytomegalovirus; IgG, immunoglobulin G; IVIg, intravenous immunoglobulin; PCR, polymerase chain reaction; PO, by mouth; QID, four times daily; TBI, total body irradiation; TID, three times daily; TMP-SMX, trimethoprim-sulfamethoxazole.

References: [1] *Biol Blood Marrow Transplant* 2009; 15(10): 1143; [2]LnID 2009; 9(2): 97; [3] National Comprehensive Cancer Network. *Prevention and Treatment of Cancer-related Infections* V.1.2008 (www.nccn.org); [4] *Biol Blood Marrow Transplant* 2006; 12(2): 138; [5] *Ann Int Med* 2003; 139: 8.

The AST Handbook of Transplant Infections, 1st edition. Edited by D. Kumar & A. Humar. © 2011 Blackwell Publishing Ltd.

43 Adult Vaccination Schedule After Solid Organ Transplant[a]

Marissa Wilck & Lindsey Baden

Recommended inactivated vaccines [1, 2]	Pre-transplant	Posttransplant[b]	Comment
Non-live vaccines			
Diptheria, tetanus and pertussis (Tdap) Diptheria and pertussis (Td)	Indicated – update prior to transplant. Give a booster dose with pertussis component (Tdap) prior to transplant	Indicated – continue booster doses with Td every 5-10 years. Administer Tdap first if not given prior to transplant	Tdap can be given ⩾ 2 years after Td
Pneumococcal a) Polysaccharide 23-valent b) Conjugated 7-,10-, or 13-valent	Indicated – transplant candidates should all receive polysaccharide vaccine	Indicated – 23-valent polysaccharide vaccine is recommended.[c] One booster after 3–5 years	Data show that conjugate vaccine priming post-transplant is not beneficial
Haemophilus influenzae type B	Consider in persons at increased risk for pneumonia	Consider in persons at increased risk for pneumonia if not previously received	No recommendations for use in adult transplant recipient
Trivalent inactivated influenza vaccine	Indicated annually	Indicated annually	Live-attenuated intranasal vaccine should not be given post-transplant
Inactivated polio	Indicated – if not previously received, give primary series	Indicated – if never previously administered and travel to high risk area give primary series	If travelling to high-risk area, give one booster dose. Live oral vaccine should not be given post-transplant
Hepatitis B[d] (a combined Hepatitis A and B vaccine is available)	Indicated – accelerated schedule should be considered to complete series prior to transplant[e] (see comment)	Indicated – if not administered pre-transplant	Higher-dose formulations may improve immune responses and are recommend prior to transplant in persons with ESRD on hemodialysis and ESLD Check anti-HBs titer 1–3 months post-vaccination (goal > 10 IU/L). Repeat vaccine series if non-response

(Continued)

The AST Handbook of Transplant Infections, 1st edition. Edited by D. Kumar & A. Humar. © 2011 Blackwell Publishing Ltd.

Recommended inactivated vaccines [1, 2]	Pre-transplant	Posttransplant[b]	Comment
Hepatitis A (a combined hepatitis A and B vaccine is available)	Indicated for all patients with ESLD, ESRD. Other medical/ behavioral indications [1]	Indicated – give primary dosages if not done prior to transplant	Consider checking titers 1–3 months after vaccination and revaccinating non-responders
Meningococcus: Conjugated (MCV4) *or* Polysaccharide (MPSV4)	Indicated for individuals at risk as per general guidelines.[f] Should receive MCV4 [1]	Indicated – if not previously received, high-risk individuals should receive MCV4 as per general guidelines [1]	If risk conditions persist and previously given MPSV4 > 5 years ago, consider revaccinating with MCV4. No comparison of the two vaccines has been made in the transplant population. MCV4 may be more immunogenic in the transplant setting
Human papillomavirus (HPV): Quadrivalent (types 6, 11, 16, 18) *or* Bivalent adjuvanted (types 16,18)	Indicated for individuals as per general guidelines [1]	Indicated as per general guidelines [1] if not previously administered	Transplant recipients with anogenital HPV are at increased risk of cervical and anogenital malignancies Immunogenicity has not been assessed in post-transplant population
Rabies	Can be given if indicated according to travel and occupational risks or post-exposure	Can be given if indicated according to travel and occupational risks or post-exposure	
Live vaccines			
MMR	Indicated. Immunize all seronegative candidates at least 1 month prior to transplant	Contraindicated	In an outbreak setting the potential benefits of vaccination may outweigh the risks.
Varicella	Indicated. Immunize all seronegative candidates at least 1 month prior to transplant	Not recommended (See comment)	Not currently recommended post transplant, although based on pediatric data some consider it safe if given in the late post transplant period.

(Continued)

(Continued)

Recommended inactivated vaccines [1, 2]	Pre-transplant	Posttransplant[b]	Comment
Varicella zoster (shingles)	Optional. Immunize seropositive candidates at least 1 month prior to transplant	Not recommended	Safety has not been determined in the pre-transplant or post-transplant setting.
Vaccinations prior to travel (see Chapter 46)			

ESLD, end-stage liver disease; ESRD, end-stage renal disease; anti-Hbs, hepatitis B surface antibody; HBV, hepatitis B virus; MMR, measles, mumps and rubella.

[a] Attempt to update all vaccines prior to any transplant.

[b] Post-transplant it is generally recommended to start immunization at 3–6 months post-transplant or when the patient is on maintenance immunosuppression. The responses are unlikely to be good before this time period. However, exceptions for earlier immunization are possible, such as during outbreaks of vaccine-preventable disease (e.g. pandemic influenza).

[c] There is no clear evidence to favor the use of the pneumococcal conjugated vaccine alone, or for priming prior to administration of the polysaccharide vaccine. The conjugate vaccine is immunogenic post-transplant and should be considered when there is documented failure of the polysaccharide vaccine. In these situations we suggest use of 13-valent vaccine rather than 7-valent.

[d] Vaccination is recommended for hepatitis B non-immune, non-infected transplant candidate. Administration of hepatitis B vaccine in candidates with active disease or recipients of organs from hepatitis B-positive donors should be individualized in consultation with an infectious diseases physician.

[e] Accelerated schedule: hepatitis B vaccine can be administered at 0, 7, and 21–28 days with a booster, if possible, at 6 months. Similarly, the combined hepatitis A and B vaccine can be used at 0, 7 and 21–28 days with a booster given at 12 months.

[f] High risk: college freshmen living in dormitories, military recruits, travel to endemic areas, participation in annual Hajj to Saudi Arabia.

References (in square brackets): [1] *MMWR* 2008; 57(53); [2] *Am J Transplantation* 2009; 9(s4): S258.

44 Adult Vaccination Schedule After Allogeneic Stem Cell Transplant

Lindsey Baden & Marissa Wilck

Recommended vaccine [1, 2]	Schedule (time post-transplant)[a]	Number of doses	Comments
Non-live vaccines			
Tetanus/diphtheria/acellular pertussis	12, 14–16 and 24 months	3	Full-dose diphtheria and pertussis (DTaP) preferred over Tdap
			Booster dose: Td every 10 years
Pneumococcal			
Conjugated 7-, 10-, or 13-valent	12, 14–16, 18 months	3	23-valent vaccine given after the conjugated in order to broaden the immune response
Polysaccharide 23-valent	24 months		Consider booster dose: 3 – 5 years
			Some recommend starting pneumococcal series early (e.g. at 3–6 months) to prevent early invasive disease; however, duration of protection may be lower with this strategy and polysaccharide booster may be less effective [3]
Haemophilus influenzae type B	12, 14–16 and 24 months	3	
Influenza	≥ 6 months post-SCT	Annually every fall	Repeat annually
			Consider vaccination starting at 4 months in high-risk settings
			Avoid the live influenza vaccine
			Novel influenza vaccines should be treated similarly when available
Inactivated polio	12, 14–16 and 24 months	3	Avoid the live vaccine
Hepatitis B	12, 14–16 and 24 months	3	Assess serological response ≥ 1 month after last dose and repeat series in non-responders. If the patient is on immunosuppressant medications, consider waiting until these are stopped before repeating series
Hepatitis A	≥ 12 months	Two doses separated by 6–12 months	Considered optional. Give according to general guidelines [1][b]

(Continued)

The AST Handbook of Transplant Infections, 1st edition. Edited by D. Kumar & A. Humar. © 2011 Blackwell Publishing Ltd.

(Continued)

Recommended vaccine [1, 2]	Schedule (time post-transplant)[a]	Number of doses	Comments
Meningococcal (conjugated vaccine)	≥ 12 months	One dose	The conjugated vaccine is preferred over the unconjugated
Human papillomavirus	≥ 12 months	Three-dose series at 0, 2, and 6 months	Follow general guidelines for women and men Immunogenicity after transplant has not been assessed
Live vaccines			
Measles, mumps, rubella (live)	≥ 24 months	One dose	Provided no significant GVHD and not on immunosuppression for at least 3 months. Some centers advocate two doses separated by ≥ 3 months
Varicella (chickenpox) (live)	At 24 months for seronegative adults	One dose	Provided no significant GVHD and not on immunosuppressive medication for at least 3 months. Some centers advocate two doses separated by ≥ 3 months
Travel or as needed			
Typhoid Vi polysaccharide (inactivated)		One dose ≥ 2 weeks prior to travel	There are no data determining safety or immunogenicity after transplant. Avoid the live typhoid vaccine
Rabies		Post-exposure prophylaxis as needed[c]	Pre-exposure prophylaxis, suggest delay of series to at least 12 months after transplant and preferably with the patient off immunosuppressive medication
Japanese B encephalitis		Prior to travel to endemic area	There are no data determining immunogenicity after transplant
Not recommended			
Varicella zoster (shingles) (live)		At this time not recommended	Higher titers of VZV than in varicella vaccine. Safety after transplant has not been determined
Yellow fever (live)		One dose	Safety not determined. Individual assessment required. Waiver may be needed for travel.
Smallpox vaccine (live)		Not recommended	In the setting of true risk individual assessment required
Oral polio (live)		Not recommended	Safer alternate vaccine available
Intranasal influenza (live)		Not recommended	Safer alternate vaccine available. Inactivated vaccine preferred for close contacts of persons early post-HSCT to avoid theoretical risk of vaccine-virus transmission.

(Continued)

Recommended vaccine [1, 2]	Schedule (time post-transplant)[a]	Number of doses	Comments
Oral typhoid (live)		Not recommended	Safer alternate vaccine available
Rotavirus (live)		Not recommended	

GVHD, graft-versus-host disease; HSCT, hematopoietic stem cell transplant; SCT, stem cell transplant; Tdap, diptheria, tetanus and pertussis; Td, diptheria and pertussis; VZV, varicella zoster virus.

[a]Vaccination of non-live vaccines is usually considered between 6 and 12 months after transplant. Decreased ability to mount an immune response early after transplant must be weighed against the risk of infection. The regimens shown above assume a 12-month start.

Patients who have active GVHD, and who have received monoclonal antibodies such as rituximab or alemtuzumab or other immunosuppressive medication will have a decreased response to vaccination, and delayed vaccination should be considered.

Some centers will perform serology at 36 months post-transplant for the following – diphtheria, tetanus, *Pneumococcus*, hepatitis B, hepatitis A, measles, mumps, rubella – and administer a booster if levels are below standard cut-offs.

Donor vaccination has been shown to improve the immunogenicity of some vaccines (e.g. 7-valent conjugate *Pneumococcus*, tetanus toxoid) but is not recommended routinely, because of practical and ethical issues.

[b]Authors practice routine administration.

[c]Give together with human rabies immunoglobulin.

Referencess: [1] *MMWR* 2008; 57(53); [2] *Bone Marrow Transplant* 2009; 44: 521; [3] *Clin Infect Dis* 2009; 48(10): 1392.

45 Immunizations After Pediatric Solid Organ Transplant and Hematopoietic Stem Cell Transplant [1–4]

Tanvi Sharma & Lynne Lewis

Vaccine	Minimum age at first dose	Type[a]	Recommended pre-transplant[b]		Recommended post-transplant[c]		Monitor titers[d]	Time to initiate vaccine and number of doses post-transplant[e] (HCT)		Comments
			SOT	HCT	SOT	HCT		Time	No. of doses	
Recommended vaccinations										
Hepatitis B	Birth	I	Yes	Yes	Yes	Yes	Yes	6–12 months	3	–
Rotavirus	6 weeks	LA	Yes[f]	Yes[f]	No/CI	No/CI	No	N/A		Do not administer first dose after 15 weeks of age. Do not administer any doses beyond 24 or 32 weeks of age depending on preparation used
Diphtheria, tetanus, acellular pertussis (DTaP)	6 weeks	I	Yes	Yes	Yes	Yes	Yes	6–12 months	3	For children <7 years of age
Tetanus, diphtheria (DT, Td)	6 weeks	I	Yes	Yes	Yes	Yes	Yes	6–12 months	3	For children >7 years of age, if they did not complete primary series with DTaP, or for booster if >5 years since last dose
Tetanus, diphtheria, acellular pertussis (Tdap)	10 years	I	Yes	Yes	Yes	Yes	Yes	6–12 months	3	For patients who have completed primary series and need booster, for adolescent/adult household contacts of young infants
Haemophilus influenzae type B (HiB)	6 weeks	I	Yes	Yes	Yes	Yes	Yes[g]	6–12 months	3	–

Vaccine	Min. age	Type					Interval	No. of doses	Comments
Pneumococcal conjugate (PCV)	6 weeks	I	Yes	Yes	Yes	Yes	3–6 months	3–4 / Age-dependent, check with national guidelines	More immunogenic than PPV23 although currently fewer serotypes in PCV. Do not use PCV7 if PCV13 available. Follow AAP guidelines regarding PCV13 administration. Administer a single dose to children 6 to 18 y.o.a. at increased risk of IPD (invasive pneumococcal disease) regardless of whether they received PCV7 or PPV23.
Pneumococcal polysaccharide (PPV23)	2 years	I	Yes	Yes	Yes	Yes	3–6 months	Age-dependent, check with national guidelines	May be used in place of fourth PCV13 dose. May produce inadequate response if administered as sole pneumococcal coverage. Administer PPV23 minimally 8 weeks or more after last PCV13 dose. Some experts recommend an interval of 16 weeks or longer between PPV23 and last PCV13 dose.
Poliovirus (IPV)	6 weeks	I	Yes	Yes	Yes	No	6–12 months	3	Do not administer live attenuated oral vaccine
Influenza – seasonal	6 months	I/LA	Yes	Yes	Yes	No	4–6 months	1–2	Do not administer intranasal live attenuated vaccine if post-transplant or contraindicated pre-transplant. Children < 9 years require two doses if receiving influenza vaccination for the first time
Measles, mumps, rubella (MMR)	6 months[h]	LA	Yes[f]	No	Yes[i]	Yes	24 months[i]	1–2	–
Varicella	12 months	LA	Yes[f]	No	Yes[i]	Yes	24 months[i]	No data	–
Hepatitis A	12 months	I	Yes	Yes	Yes	Yes	6–12 months	2	Should be administered routinely for patients in whom transplant is anticipated. There are no data on efficacy post-HCT
Meningococcal (conjugate vaccine: MCV)	2 years	I	Yes	Yes	Yes	No	6–12 months	1	–

(Continued)

(Continued)

Vaccine	Minimum age at first dose	Type[a]	Recommended pre-transplant[b]		Recommended post-transplant[c]		Monitor titers[d]	Time to initiate vaccine and number of doses post-transplant[e] HCT		Comments
			SOT	HCT	SOT	HCT		Time	No. of doses	
Human papilloma-virus (HPV)	9 years	I	Yes	Yes	Yes	Yes	No	6 months	Series	No data on efficacy post HCT
Outbreak/exposure/situational vaccines										
Rabies	Birth	I	Yes	Yes	Yes	Yes	No	N/A		Recommended only for post-exposure prophylaxis
Smallpox	N/A	LA	No	No	No/CI	No/CI	No	N/A		Household members of immunocompromised patients should not receive vaccine; not indicated except in specific situations
Bacillus Calmette-Guérin (BCG)	Birth	LA	No	No	No	No	No	N/A		Not indicated except in specific situations
Anthrax	N/A	I	No	No	No	No	No	N/A		Not indicated except in specific situations
Travel vaccines (see Chapter 46)										

CI, contraindicated; HCT, hematopoietic cell transplant; I, inactivated; LA, live attenuated; N/A, not applicable.

[a]Household members of SOTs and HCTs:
– OPV (not available in US) and smallpox vaccines contraindicated
– MMR, varicella zoster virus and rotavirus recommended
– All household members should be fully immunized against poliovirus, measles, mumps, rubella, varicella, influenza and hepatitis A.

[b]Follow Centers for Disease Control childhood vaccination schedules. Accelerated vaccination schedule may be implemented prior to transplant to maximize number of doses received.

[c]Whenever possible, for SOT the complete vaccination series should be administered prior to transplantation. Vaccines that may be safe for administration post-transplantation may not be sufficiently immunogenic.

[d] Titers: if there is an available test for a known antibody correlate of protection, specific serum antibody titers should be determined 4–6 weeks after immunization to assess immune response and guide further immunization and management of future exposures.

[e] Where data exist, number of doses, followed by titers where available, are recommended for HCT per published HCT guidelines. For SOT, a complete series should be completed (including pre-transplant doses) and titers drawn where available.

[f] Administer pre-transplant only if there is an anticipated minimum 4-week interval before planned listing for transplant and if there is no pre-transplant immunosuppression such as chemotherapy.

[g] Where available.

[h] May be administered as early as 6 months of age in patients in whom transplant is anticipated prior to 12 months of age. However, the immunogenicity of vaccine administered at 6 months of age is unknown.

[i] May be considered in patients > 24 months post-HCT, with no graft-versus-host disease, and who are off immunosuppression for at least 3 months.

References (in square brackets): [1] Am J Transplantation 2009: 9(s4): S258; [2] AAP Redbook 2009; [3] Bone Marrow Transplant 2009; 44: 521; [4] Am J Transplantation 2008; 8: 9. [5] American Academy of Pediatrics Committee on Infectious Diseases. Policy statement recommendations for the prevention of streptococcus pneumoniae infections in infants and children: Use of 13-valent pneumococcal conjugate vaccine (PCV 13) and pneumococcal polysaccharide vaccine (PPV23). Pediatrics 2010; 126(1): 1–5.

46 Recommendations for Travel-related Vaccinations and Medications for Transplant Travelers

Camille N. Kotton

46.1 Recommendations for travel-related vaccinations for transplant travelers

Vaccine	Adults	Children
Hepatitis A	Recommended for travel to endemic regions; consider using IVIg or intramuscular Ig for more immunocompromised patients	Recommended per CDC guidelines, minimum age for first dose 12 months
Hepatitis B	Recommended when indicated	Recommended per CDC guidelines, at birth
Meningococcal conjugate	Recommended when indicated	Recommended per CDC guidelines, minimum age for first dose 2 years
Rabies	Recommended when indicated	Recommended when indicated, any age
Japanese encephalitis	Recommended when indicated	Recommended when indicated, minimum for first dose 12 months
Inactivated polio (IPV)	Recommended when indicated	Recommended when indicated, minimum age 6 weeks
Oral polio (OPV)[a]	Contraindicated in patients/family members	Contraindicated in patients/family members
Salmonella typhi (Typhim Vi)	Recommended when indicated	Recommended when indicated for ages > 2 years
S. typhi Ty21a (Vivotif)[a]	Contraindicated	Contraindicated
Bacille Calmette-Guérin[a]	Contraindicated	Contraindicated
Yellow fever[a]	Contraindicated	Contraindicated

CDC, Centers for Disease Control; IVIg, intravenous immunoglobulin.
[a]Live, attenuated.

Referencess: [1] http://www.cdc.gov/vaccines/recs/schedules/adult-schedule.htm; [2] http://wwwnc.cdc.gov/travel/yellow-book/2010/chapter-8/immunocompromised-traveler.aspx; [3] *Am J Transplantation* 2005; 5(1): 8; [4] *Am J Transplantation* 2009; (s4): 273.

46.2 Travel-related medications, adult dosages, and duration

	Dose	Duration	Change for reduced GFR	Change for hepatic dysfunction
Diarrhea treatment				
Ciprofloxacin	500 mg BID	For 3–7 days	Yes	No
Levofloxacin	500 mg/day	For 3–7 days	Yes	No
Azithromycin	500 mg/day	For 3–7 days	Caution if CrCl < 10 mL/min	No
Malaria prophylaxis				
Atovaquone-proguanil	Atovaquone/proguanil 250 mg/100 mg/day	Start 1–2 days prior to entering a malaria-endemic area; continue daily throughout the stay and for 7 days after leaving malarious area	Not for mild to moderate renal impairment; avoid if severe renal impairment (CrCl < 30 mL/min)	No dosage adjustment required in mild-to-moderate hepatic impairment There are no data for use in severe hepatic impairment
Doxycycline	100 mg/day	Start 1–2 days before entering a malaria-endemic area; continue daily during the stay and for 7 days after leaving malarious area	No	No
Mefloquine	250 mg/week	Begin 1–2 weeks before, arrival in endemic area; continue weekly during travel and for 4 weeks after leaving endemic area	No	Half-life may be prolonged and plasma levels may be higher
Chloroquine	500 mg/week (300 mg base), weekly	Begin 1–2 weeks prior to exposure; continue for 4 weeks after leaving endemic area	Administer 50% of dose if CrCl < 10 mL/min	No dosage adjustment required
Altitude illness prophylaxis				
Acetazolamide	125–250 mg BID	Begin two days before ascending and continue until two days after completing ascent	Yes	No

BID, twice daily; CrCl, creatinine clearance; GFR, glomerular filtration rate.

46.3 Interactions between transplant and travel-related medications[a]

	Calcineurin inhibitors (CNIs)	Trimethoprim/sulfamethoxazole
Acetazolamide (Diamox®)	May increase CNI levels	
Artemether/lumefantrine (Coartem®)	May enhance the QT-prolonging effect of CNI	
Atovaquone/proguanil (Malarone®)		May increase risk of bone marrow toxicity
Azithromycin (Zithromax®)	May increase CNI levels	
Chloroquine (Aralen®)	May increase CNI levels	May enhance the QT-prolonging effect of CNI
Doxycycline	May increase CNI levels	
Mefloquine (Lariam®)	May increase CNI levels	May enhance the QT-prolonging effect of CNI
Primaquine	May increase CNI levels	
Sulfadoxine/pyrimethamine (Fansidar®)	May reduce CNI levels	May increase risk of bone marrow toxicity

[a]Significant interactions of travel medicines and azathioprine, mycophenolate mofetil, and corticosteroids have not been reported; significant interactions of transplant medicines and levofloxacin, diphenoxylate hydrochloride and atropine sulfate tablets or loperamide have not been reported; there are minimal data available.

Adapted from MicroMedex® DrugReax® Interactive Drug Interactions and Lexi-Comp Online™ Interaction Analysis

47 Safe Living Strategies for Transplant Patients

Julia Garcia-Diaz & Shannon Bergeron

Recommendations	Comments/associated pathogens
Prevention of infections transmitted by direct contact	
• Handwashing in all settings (soap and water preferable but hand rubs are acceptable)	*Salmonella*, rotavirus, *Staphylococcus* sp., *Sporothrix*, enteric pathogens, *Pseudomonas* sp., *Mycobacteria* sp.
– before eating or preparing food	
– before and after touching mucous membranes	
– after touching or cleaning up pets or other animals	
– after gardening or touching plants or soil	
– after changing diapers (this activity should be performed by a family member whenever possible)	
– after touching items contaminated with human or animal feces	
– after touching secretions and excretions	
– before and after touching wounds	
• Avoid walking barefooted	
• Use insect repellent when outside for long periods	
• Wear gloves whenever gardening	
• Avoid percutaneous exposures: IV drug use, body piercing and tattoos	
Prevention of respiratory infections	
• Handwashing	Rhinoviruses, influenza A & B, other viral respiratory pathogens
– before and after touching mucous membranes	
• Avoid sick contacts and wear mask if contact is unavoidable	*Streptococcus pneumoniae*, *Haemophilus influenza*, *Mycobacterium tuberculosis*, *Chlamydia* sp.
• Avoid crowds (shopping malls, subways, elevators) especially during periods of enhanced immunosuppression	*Aspergillus*, endemic fungi (*Cryptococcus*, *Histoplasma*, *Coccidioides*, *Blastomyces*)
• Avoid tobacco smoke	*Nocardia*
• Avoid marijuana smoking	
• Avoid contact with people at high risk for exposure to tuberculosis (homeless shelters, jails, etc.)	
• Avoid construction sites, excavations and other dust-laden environments (areas with high concentration of mold spores)	
• Avoid exposure to plant and soil aerosols, pigeon and other bird droppings, chicken coops and caves	
• Avoid cleaning of bird cages and cat litter pans	
• Avoid gardening for first year after transplant, or, if unavoidable, wear masks and gloves	
• Pneumococcal and influenza vaccinations up to date	

(Continued)

The AST Handbook of Transplant Infections, 1st edition. Edited by D. Kumar & A. Humar. © 2011 Blackwell Publishing Ltd.

Recommendations	Comments/associated pathogens
Water safety	
• Avoid consumption of untreated tap water (beware of ice, fountain beverages served at restaurants, bars, sporting events, etc.)	*Cryptosporidium* (resistant to chlorine), *Giardia*, bacterial coliforms, *Leptospira*, *Legionella*, *Mycobacteria* sp., *Pseudomonas* sp.
• If untreated tap water is unavoidable, boil water for 1 minute or drink bottled water[a]	
• Avoid drinking water from wells	
• Avoid consumption of water while participating in water activities in lakes, rivers, swimming pools, and at amusement parks	
• Avoid using hot tubs	
• Clean standing water in the home or basement promptly	
• Avoid drinking tap water when traveling to countries with poor sanitation	
• Clean wounds/abrasions incurred while bathing in the ocean or fresh water (rivers, lakes, etc)	
Food safety	
• Avoid soft cheeses (feta, brie, camembert) or cheese made with unpasteurized milk	*Listeria*, *Escherichia coli* 0157:H7, *Salmonella*, *Brucella*, *Yersinia*, and *Cryptosporidium*, *Vibrio* sp., hepatitis A, other viruses that cause gastroenteritis
• Avoid drinking or eating food made with unpasteurized milk, or drinking unpasteurized fruit or vegetable juice/cider	
• Avoid consumption of raw or undercooked eggs (cake and cookie batter, Caesar salad dressing, mayonnaise or Hollandaise sauce)	
• Avoid all raw or undercooked meat, poultry, or seafood (fish, oysters, clams, mussels)	
• Avoid cross-contamination when preparing food	
• Avoid open salad bars	
• Thoroughly wash and/or peel fruits and vegetables	
• Reheat leftovers to steaming hot	
• Avoid food left at room temperature for long periods of time	
Animal contact	
• Handwashing	*Toxoplasma gondii*, *Cryptosporidium*, *Salmonella*, *Campylobacter*, *Bartonella*, lymphocytic choriomeningitis virus, rabies
– wash hands after handling animals	
– wash hands after handling/cleaning cages, litter boxes	
• Transplant recipients who work with animals should avoid working during periods of maximal immunosuppression	
• Avoid contact with animals with diarrhea	
• Avoid stray animals	
• Avoid animal bites or scratches	
• Avoid contact with rodents, kittens, reptiles (snakes, iguanas, lizards, and turtles), chicks, and ducklings	
• Avoid contact with monkeys	
• Wear gloves to clean aquariums or have someone else do cleaning	
• Avoid cleaning bird cages, bird feeders and litter boxes	
• Avoid handling animal feces	

(Continued)

(*Continued*)

Recommendations	Comments/associated pathogens
Safe sexual practices	
• Always use latex condoms during sexual contact outside of long-term monogamous relationships • Avoid feces exposure during sexual activity	Cytomegalovirus, hepatitis B and C, HIV, human papillomavirus, herpes simplex virus, other sexually transmitted diseases
Travel safety	

• During travel in developing countries (see 'Food safety' above)
  – avoid consumption of tap water, ice and beverages made with tap water
  – avoid fresh fruit juices
  – avoid unpasteurized milk and dairy products
  – avoid raw, unpeeled fruits and vegetables
  – avoid raw or undercooked meat, poultry, seafood, or eggs
• Transplant recipient should always:
  – seek pre-travel medical advice
  – ingest fruits and vegetables that can be peeled
  – ingest steaming hot foods
  – drink bottled and processed drinks
  – tap water can be boiled (1 minute) or disinfected with iodine or portable filters
  – avoid street vendor food
• Recommend use of hats, sunglasses, protective clothing, and sunblock with UVA and UVB protection
• Antibiotics should be given to take in case of diarrhea
• Prescribe malaria prophylaxis based on travel itinerary
• Take a sufficient supply of medications for the period of travel as well as a medication list
• Immunization status should be evaluated and updated
• Administer vaccines based on anticipated travel itinerary
• Live virus vaccines should be avoided
• See also 'Water safety' above
	Cryptosporidium, *Salmonella*, *Brucella*, *Vibrio* sp. bacterial coliforms, *Giardia*, *Strongyloides*, malaria

[a]International Bottled Water Association (information regarding bottle water) (1-703-683-5213 or http://www.bottled-water.org).

Suggested websites: American Society of Transplantation (patient education brochures)(http://www.a-s-t.org); Centers for Disease Control (updated travel advisories) (http://www.cdc.gov)

References: [1] *Am J Transplantation* 2009; 9(s4): S252; [2] *Am J Transplantation* 2005; 5: 8; [3] *Am J Transplantation* 2009; 9(s4): S3; [4] *MMWR Recomm Rep* 2000; 49 (RR-10):1.

NSF standard 053 for cryptosporidial cyst removal can be obtained by contacting the NSF International consumer line: 1-800-673-8010.

PART V
Post-transplant Medications and Drug Interactions

48 Common Immunosuppressive Drugs, Mechanisms of Action, Side-effects, and Other Interactions

Daniel Kaul

Drug	Mechanism of Action	Selected adverse effects	Selected drug interactions/comments
Agents commonly used for maintenance immunosuppression			
Calcineurin inhibitors (CNIs) Tacrolimus (Tac) (Prograf®) Cyclosporine (CsA) (Sandimmune®) Cyclosporine (CsA) Modified (Neoral®, Gengraf®)	Inhibition of early activation of T lymphocytes	CsA and Tac: nephrotoxicity, hyperkalemia, hypomagnesemia, hyperuricemia, nausea, HUS/TTP (rare) Tac > CsA: neurotoxicity (headache, tremors), PRES, glucose intolerance CsA > Tac: hypertension, hyperlipidemia CsA only: gingival hyperplasia, hirsutism Tac only: alopecia	Increase CNI levels: antifungal azoles[a], protease inhibitors, macrolide antibiotics[b], calcium channel blockers[c], grapefruit juice Decrease CNI levels: rifampin > rifabutin, sirolimus(Tac only), antiseizure medications[d], St John's wort CNIs increase levels: statins, sirolimus(CsA only) Synergistic effects: aminoglycosides, amphotericin, NSAIDs – nephrotoxicity
Anti-metabolites Mycophenolate mofetil (MMF) (CellCept®) Mycophenolate sodium (MPS) (myfortic®) Azathioprine (AZA) (Imuran®)	Interference with nucleotide synthesis and prevention of T- and B-cell proliferation	MMF/MPS > AZA: GI toxicity (nausea, vomiting, abdominal pain, diarrhea) AZA and MMF/MPS: bone marrow suppression AZA only: rash, cholestatic jaundice	Synergistic effects: valganciclovir, TMP-SMX – bone marrow suppression Increase AZA activity/toxicity: allopurinol Decrease MMF/MPS absorption: cholestyramine, antacids
mTOR inhibitors Sirolimus (SRL) (Rapamune®) Everolimus (EVL) (Zortress®)	Inhibition of T-cell activation and proliferation signaling	Diarrhea/nausea, bone marrow suppression, impaired wound healing, interstitial pneumonitis, hyperlipidemia, mouth ulcers, lymphocele, HUS/TTP (rare; with CNI), skin rash, acne, peripheral edema	Increased SRL/EVL levels: antifungal azoles[a], protease inhibitors, macrolide antibiotics[b], calcium channel blockers[c], cyclosporine, grapefruit juice Decrease SRL/EVL levels: rifampin, rifabutin, antiseizure medications[d], St John's wort

(Continued)

129

(Continued)

Drug	Mechanism of Action	Selected adverse effects	Selected drug interactions/ comments
Corticosteroids (used at higher doses for rejection)	Multiple anti-inflammatory effects including suppression of leukocyte migration	Glucose intolerance, edema, hypokalemia, muscle weakness, avascular necrosis, acne, hypertension, hyperlipidemia, peptic ulcers, impaired wound healing, mood swings, psychosis	Synergistic effects: NSAIDs – increased risk of GI bleeding

Agents commonly used for acute rejection and/or induction of immunosuppression

Rabbit anti-thymocyte globulin (Thymoglobulin®)	Polyclonal antibody resulting in prolonged depletion of T-cells	Fevers/chills (infusion-related), leukopenia, thrombocytopenia, aseptic meningitis, serum sickness, skin rash, anaphylaxis (rare)	No known significant drug interactions Premedication recommended Use: induction, rejection
Muromonab-CD3, OKT3 (Orthoclone OKT® 3)	Anti-CD3 monoclonal antibody resulting in T-cell depletion	Anaphylaxis (rare), cytokine release syndrome (mild flu-like to multisystem: pulmonary, edema, fevers), neurological (aseptic meningitis, seizures), leukopenia	No known significant drug interactions Premedication recommended Manufacturer has discontinued, or is in the process of discontinuing, North American production. Supplies expected to be diminished by late 2010/early 2011
Alemtuzumab (Campath®)	Anti-CD52 monoclonal antibody resulting in prolonged depletion of mononuclear cells	Bone marrow suppression, infusion reactions including anaphylaxis	No known significant drug interactions Premedication recommended Use: Induction Rejection
IL-2 Receptor antagonists Basiliximab (Simulect®) Daclizumab (Zenapax®)*	Anti-CD25 monoclonal antibody that prevents IL-2 activation of T-lymphocytes	Hypersensitivity reactions (rare)	No known significant drug interactions No premedication recommended Use: Induction
Rituximab (Rituxan®)	Anti-CD20 monoclonal antibody resulting in B-cell depletion	Hypersensitivity reactions (rare), hypotension, infusion reactions, pancytopenia	No known significant drug interactions Premedication recommended Use: induction (rare), humoral rejection

HUS, hemolytic uremic syndrome; IL, interleukin; mTOR, mammalian target of rapamycin; NSAIDS, non-steroidal anti-inflammatory drugs; PRES, posterior reversible encephalopathy syndrome; TMP-SMX, trimethoprim- sulfamethoxazole; TTP, thrombotic thrombocytopenic purpura

[a]Ketoconazole, , voriconazole, itraconazole, posaconazole, fluconazole, clotrimazole.
[b]Erythromycin, clarithromycin.
[c]Diltiazem , verapamil, nicardipine.
[d]Carbamazepine, phenobarbital, phenytoin.

References: [1] *New Engl J Med* 2004; 351: 2715; [2] *Clin Infect Dis* 2009; 48: 772; [3] *Crit Rev Oncol Hematol* 2005; 56: 23.

49 Infectious Risks Associated with Anti-thymocyte Globulin (ATG, Thymoglobulin)

Steven D. Burdette

Mechanism of action: Anti-thymocyte globulin (ATG) is a polyclonal antibody that induces dose-dependent depletion of T cells while also having some effect on B cells. It also interferes with dendritic cells, regulatory T cells, and natural killer cell functions. The degree of T-cell depletion is based on total dose administered and the duration of therapy.

Duration of effect: Profound CD3 lymphopenia may last up to 1 year.

	Risk	Impact on laboratory monitoring	Impact on prophylaxis	Comments
Bacterial infections	Unclear impact	Aggressive microbiologic evaluation for febrile transplant recipients who have received ATG	No impact	Reported bacterial complications include UTI, wound infections, pneumonia [1]. Not associated with *Nocardia* infection [2]
BK virus	Increased risk of infection, especially with higher doses of ATG administration [3,4]	Consider more frequent screening (monthly rather than quarterly)	N/A	Due to prolonged CD3 lymphopenia, may have prolonged BK viremia compared with other agents (such as IL-2R antagonists)
CMV	Increased risk of infection [5]	If pre-emptive protocol followed, consider extended duration of monitoring. Consider screening for CMV reactivation after completing prophylaxis	Consider extended prophylaxis to 6 months, especially in D+/R−	CD3 lymphopenia can last for up to 1 year, and may impact the incidence of infection after completion of prophylaxis
EBV/PTLD	Possible increased risk, especially EBV D+/R−, although data are mixed [6, 7]	Active screening for EBV viremia if EBV D+/R−	Consider antiviral prophylaxis in D+/R− patients	Consider avoiding ATG in EBV D+/R−, if possible

(Continued)

The AST Handbook of Transplant Infections, 1st edition. Edited by D. Kumar & A. Humar. © 2011 Blackwell Publishing Ltd.

(Continued)

	Risk	Impact on laboratory monitoring	Impact on prophylaxis	Comments
Fungal infections	No increased risk with induction [1, 4] Increased risk with rejection therapy	If known exposure to endemic fungus[a], routine screening is likely indicated	If known exposure to endemic fungi, prophylaxis for 3–12 months is indicated	Associated with false-positive *Histoplasma* urine antigens if older assays utilized [9, 10]
HCV/HBV	Accelerated HCV replication but no increased rate of hepatic graft injury [11] Not associated with poor outcomes with HCV+ renal transplant patients [12]	Consider routine viral load monitoring in those known to have positive viremia Consider monitoring for reactivation of viremia in recipients with negative viral loads prior to transplant	Consider HBV prophylaxis for anti-HBc or HbsAg-positive patients even if viral loads are undetectable	Data are lacking regarding progression of HBV infection associated with ATG
Pneumocystis	Increased risk of infection without appropriate prophylaxis [13]	N/A	Minimum of 6–12 months of prophylaxis Consider prolonged prophylaxis in heart and/or lung recipients	Risk is alleviated with proper prophylaxis

CMV, cytomegalovirus; D+/R–, donor positive/recipient negative; EBV, Epstein–Barr virus; anti-HBc, hepatitis B core antibody; HBsAg, hepatitis B surface antigen; HBV, hepatitis B virus; HCV, hepatitis C virus; IL-2R, interleukin-2R; PTLD, post-transplant lymphoproliferative disorder; UTI, urinary tract infection.

[a]Endemic fungi include but are not limited to histoplasmosis, blastomycosis, and coccidioidomycosis.

References (in square brackets): [1] *Clin Transplant* 2003; 17: 69; [2] *Clin Infect Dis* 2007; 44(10): 1307; [3] *Transplantation* 2008; 86: 521; [4] *American Transplant Congress* 2008, abst 390; [5] *Transplantation* 2003; 75(6): 844; [6] *Liver Transpl* 2007; 13: 1039; [7] *Transplant Infect Dis* 2001; 3: 203; [8] *Transpl Int* 2007; 20 (5): 447; [9] *Transplant Infect Dis* 2004; 6: 23; [10] *Transplant Infect Dis* 2006; 8: 219; [11] *Clin Infect Dis* 2009; 48(6): 772; [12] *Am J Transplantation* 2005; 5: 1452; [13] *Am J Transplantation* 2002; 2: 48.

50 Infectious Risks Associated with Alemtuzumab (Campath)

Steven D. Burdette

Mechanism of action: Lymphoid depletion (including pan T-cell depletion) decreases global immune activity, leading to a lower anti-donor response.

Duration of effect: B lymphocytes return within 3–12 months but CD4 lymphocytes may remain $< 100/\mu L$ for 18–24 months.

	Risk	Impact on laboratory monitoring	Impact on prophylaxis	Comments
Bacterial infections	No increased risk, including *Streptococcus*, *Listeria*, *Nocardia* or MAC (common pathogens in AIDS) [1]	Aggressive microbiologic evaluation for febrile transplant recipients who have received alemtuzumab	No impact	
BK virus	Increased risk as compared with IL-2R antagonists or no induction [2] but similar to ATG [3]	Consider more frequent screening (monthly rather than quarterly)	N/A	Due to prolonged CD4 lymphopenia, may have prolonged BK viremia compared with other agents (such as IL-2R antagonists)
CMV	Increased risk as compared with IL-2R antagonists [4] but likely similar to ATG	Consider either prolonged pre-emptive protocols or screening for reactivation after completion of prophylaxis	Consider extended prophylaxis to 6 months or longer, especially in D+/R–; failure of prophylaxis has been reported	CD3/4 lymphopenia can last over 1 year, and may impact incidence of infection after completion of prophylaxis
EBV/PTLD	Likely increased risk but data are mixed and long-term data are lacking	EBV D+/R– patients should be monitored for EBV viremia	Consider antiviral prophylaxis in D+/R– patients	Recent data show no increased risk in kidney or pancreas kidney
Fungal infections	No increased risk when used for induction. Significant increased risk when used for rejection.	If exposure to endemic fungus[a], routine screening likely indicated	If exposure to endemic fungi, prophylaxis for 6–12 months is indicated	Most infections occurred within 3 months of therapy. Not associated with zygomycosis infection

(Continued)

The AST Handbook of Transplant Infections, 1st edition. Edited by D. Kumar & A. Humar. © 2011 Blackwell Publishing Ltd.

(*Continued*)

	Risk	Impact on laboratory monitoring	Impact on prophylaxis	Comments
HCV/HBV	No benefit over conventional induction treatment for liver transplant with potential for increased complications, including systemic infection [5]	Consider routine viral load monitoring in patients known to have positive viremia Consider monitoring for reactivation of viremia in recipients with negative viral loads prior to transplant	Consider HBV prophylaxis for anti-HBc or HbsAg-positive patients even if viral loads are undetectable	Data lacking regarding progression of HBV infection associated with alemtuzumab
Miscellaneous infections	*Balamuthia* meningitis and *Toxoplasma* pneumonia have been reported	N/A	TMP-SMX prophylaxis preferred for PCP due to protection against *Toxoplasmosis*	
Pneumocystis	Prolonged risk due to T-cell depletion	N/A	Minimum of 6–12 months' prophylaxis Consider more prolonged prophylaxis in heart and/or lung recipients	Risk is alleviated with proper prophylaxis

AIDS, acquired immune deficiency syndrome; ATG, anti-thymocyte globulin; CMV, cytomegalovirus; D+/R–, donor positive/recipient negative; EBV, Epstein–Barr virus; anti-HBc, hepatitis B core antibody; HBsAg, hepatitis B surface antigen; HBV, hepatitis B virus; HCV, hepatitis C virus; IL-2R, interleukin-2R; MAC, *Mycobacterium avium* complex; PCP, *Pneumocystis carinii* pneumonia; PTLD, post-transplant lymphoproliferative disorder; TMP-SMX, trimethoprim- sulfamethoxazole.
aEndemic fungi include but are not limited to histoplasmosis, blastomycosis, and coccidioidomycosis.

References (in square brackets): [1] *Clin Infect Dis* 2007; 44(10): 1307; [2] *Transplantation* 2006; 82(3): 382; [3] *Transplantation* 2009; 87(4): 525; [4] *Clin Infect Dis* 2007; 44(2): 204; [5] *Transplantation* 2004; 78(7): 966.

51 Infectious Risks Associated with IL-2R Antagonist [Basiliximab (Simulect) and Daclizumab (Zenapax)]

Steven D. Burdette

Mechanism of action: Interleukin-2 (IL-2) antagonist saturate the IL-2 receptors and prevent T cells from replication and also from activating the B cells, which are responsible for the production of antibodies.

Duration of effect: Less than 3 months

	Risk	Impact on laboratory Monitoring	Impact on prophylaxis	Comments
Bacterial infections	No increased risk during induction [1]	No impact	No impact	–
BK virus	No increased risk	Standard BK screening protocols	N/A	Potentially more rapid viral clearance with appropriate intervention as compared with other induction agents
CMV	No increased risk during induction [2, 3]	No impact	No impact	–
EBV/PTLD	No increased risk [1, 3]	Standard EBV screening protocols for EBV D+/R– SOT recipients	No impact	–
Fungal infections	No increased risk [4]	No impact	No impact	–
HCV/HBV	Data are mixed, demonstrating both increased risk and no risk of recurrent HCV infection	Standard monitoring	N/A for HCV Follow standard protocols for HBV prophylaxis	No data available for HBV-infected patients
Pneumocystis	No increased risk [4, 6, 7]	N/A	No impact	–

CMV, cytomegalovirus; D+/R–, donor positive/recipient negative; EBV, Epstein–Barr virus; HBV, hepatitis B virus; HCV, hepatitis C virus; PTLD, post-transplant lymphoproliferative disorder; SOT, solid organ transplant.

References (in square brackets): [1] *Am J Transplantation* 2002; 2: 48; [2] *New England J Med* 2005; 352: 2705; [3] *Lancet* 1997; 350: 1193; [4] *New England J Med* 2006; 355: 1967; [5] *Transplantation* 2001; 72: 1915; [6] *J Heart Lung Transplant* 2005; 24: 296; [7] *J Heart Lung Transplant* 2007; 26: 693.

The AST Handbook of Transplant Infections, 1st edition. Edited by D. Kumar & A. Humar. © 2011 Blackwell Publishing Ltd.

52 Infectious Risks Associated With Rituximab (Rituxan)

Steven D. Burdette

Mechanism of action: Depletes CD20+ B-cells thus affecting humoral immunity and does not affect the T cell immune response.

Duration of effect: Recovered B cells may lack the TNF receptor for up to 2 years.

	Risk	Impact on laboratory monitoring	Impact on prophylaxis	Comments
Bacterial infections	No increased risk [1]	No impact	No impact	–
BK virus	No increased risk [1]	No impact	N/A	–
CMV	No increased risk compared to other regimens [1, 2]	No impact	No impact	Potential increased risk if used for rejection, though data are variable [3]
EBV/PTLD	No increased risk, potentially protective [4]	No impact	No impact	Often used as therapy for CD20-positive tumors
Fungal infections	No apparent increased risk [1] although data conflicting	No impact	No impact	Higher risk of fungal infection reported in one study [5]
HCV/HBV	Increased risk for HBV reactivation [6] There are a lack of data regarding HCV	Monitor for HBV reactivation	Consider HBV prophylaxis when anti-Hbc-positive	Available data mostly from non-transplant patients
Miscellaneous infections	Increased risk for JC virus infection (cause of PML) No association with TB [7]	N/A	N/A	–
Pneumocystis	No increased risk (no impact on T cells)	No impact	Prophylaxis only if other high-risk agents administered	Case reports of PCP infection in the oncologic population

CMV, cytomegalovirus; DEBV, Epstein–Barr virus; anti-HBc, hepatitis B core antibody; HBV, hepatitis B virus; HCV, hepatitis C virus; PCP, *Pneumocystis carinii* pneumonia; PML, progressive multifocal leukoencephalopathy; PTLD, post-transplant lymphoproliferative disorder.

References (in square brackets): [1] *Transplantation* 2009; 87(9): 1325; [2] *Transpl Int* 2009; 22(10): 961; [3] *Transplantation* 2007; 83: 1277; [4] *Transplantation* 2008; 85(9): 1290; [5] *Am J Transplantation* 2010; 10: 89; [6] *Expert Opin Drug Saf* 2005; 5: 599; [7] *Ann Rheum Dis* 2009; 68: 25.

The AST Handbook of Transplant Infections, 1st edition. Edited by D. Kumar & A. Humar. © 2011 Blackwell Publishing Ltd.

53 Drug Interactions Between Antimicrobial Agents and Common Immunosuppressive Drugs Used in Transplantation

Christian Garzoni

Antimicrobial drug	Interaction with:	Interactions/required dose adjustment
Antibacterial agents		
Fluoroquinolones		
Ciprofloxacin	CsA	Potential for mild increase in CsA levels. Not usually clinically significant
Macrolides		
Erythromycin	CsA, Tac, SRL , EVL	Known significant increase in CsA, Tac, SRL and EVL levels. TDM required
Clarithromycin	CsA, Tac, SRL, EVL	Known significant increase in CsA, Tac, SRL and EVL levels. TDM required
Azithromycin	CsA	Potential for mild increase in CsA levels. TDM recommended
Aminoglycosides		
Gentamicin, tobramycin, amikacin	CsA, Tac	Increased nephrotoxicity, avoid combination
Miscellaneous		
Rifampin	CsA, Tac, SRL, EVL	Known significant decrease in CsA, Tac, SRL, EVL levels. Avoid combination if possible. TDM is required. Consider rifabutin as an alternative (less severe induction)
	MMF	Possible moderate decrease in MMF exposure, mechanism unknown. Avoid combination if possible
Quinupristin/dalfopristin	CsA, Tac	Possible moderate increase in CsA levels. TDM recommended
TMP-SMX	MMF, Aza	When used together, potential for synergistic increase in bone marrow toxicity
Vancomycin	CsA, Tac	Possible increased nephrotoxicity
Antifungals		
Amphotericin B deoxycholate	CsA, Tac	Increased nephrotoxicity, avoid combination
Liposomal amphotericin B formulations	CsA, Tac	Increased nephrotoxicity, less profound as seen with amphotericin B deoxycholate

(Continued)

(Continued)

Antimicrobial drug	Interaction with:	Interactions/required dose adjustment
Echinocandins		
Caspofungin	CsA	Possible increase in caspofungin exposure, clinical relevance not clear. Possible increase in liver enzymes in healthy volunteers but not shown in transplant patients
	Tac	Possible decrease in Tac levels. May not be clinically significant. TDM recommended
Micafungin	SRL	Possible increase in SRL levels. May not be clinically significant. TDM recommended
Anidulafungin	CsA	Possible increase in anidulafungin exposure, clinical relevance unknown
Azole antifungal		Inhibitors of CYP450 metabolism. Inhibitory potential: ketoconazole > itraconazole ≈ voriconazole > posaconazole > fluconazole
Ketoconazole	CsA,Tac, SRL, EVL	Known significant increase in CsA, Tac, SRL and EVL levels. TDM required. Suggested dose reductions: CsA (70–80%), Tac (50–60%), SRL (80–90%), EVL (unknown minimum 50%)
Itraconazole	CsA,Tac, SRL, EVL	Known significant increase in CsA, Tac, SRL and EVL levels. TDM required. Suggested dose reductions: CsA (50–60%), Tac (50–60%), SRL and EVL (unknown, minimum 40%)
Voriconazole	CsA,Tac, SRL, EVL	Known significant increase in CsA, Tac, SRL and EVL levels. TDM required. Suggested dose reductions: CsA (50%), Tac (66%), SRL (contraindicated though reductions of 90% have been reported), EVL (unknown, minimum 40%)
Posaconazole	CsA,Tac, SRL, EVL	Known significant increase in CsA, Tac, SRL and EVL levels. Use of posaconazole with sirolimus is contraindicated. TDM required. Suggested dose reductions: CsA (up to 30%), Tac (75–80%), EVL (unknown, minimum 40%)
Fluconazole	CsA,Tac, SRL, EVL	Known significant increase in CsA, Tac, SRL and EVL levels. TDM required. Suggested dose reductions: CsA (20–50%), Tac (40%), SRL (50–70%) and EVL (unknown, minimum 40%)
Antivirals		
Acyclovir/valacyclovir	MMF	Possible increase risk of acyclovir toxicity in the setting of renal insufficiency when co-administered with MMF
Ganciclovir/valganciclovir	Aza, MMF	Increased risk of cytopenia
Foscarnet	CsA, Tac	Probable increased nephrotoxicity
Cidofovir	CsA, Tac	Probable increased nephrotoxicity
Highly active antiretroviral therapy (HAART)		Significant drug–drug interactions exist with protease inhibitor containing HAART regimens. Collaboration with an infectious diseases-HIV specialist and transplant pharmacist is highly recommended
Nucleoside reverse transcriptase inhibitors (NRTIs)		
AZT, abacavir	MMF	MMF undergoes glucuronidation like AZT and abacavir. Potential for increased risk of mitochondrial toxicity when used together. TDM recommended

(Continued)

(*Continued*)

Antimicrobial drug	Interaction with:	Interactions/required dose adjustment
Tenofovir	CsA, Tac	Potential for synergistic nephrotoxicity, monitoring of renal function is recommended
Protease inhibitors		
Atazanavir, darunavir, fosamprenavir, indinavir, lopinavir/ritonavir, nelfinavir, ritonavir, saquinavir, tipranavir	CsA, Tac, SRL, EVL	Known significant increase in CsA, Tac, SRL and EVL levels. TDM required. Suggested dose modification when used in combination with PIs: CsA (15–25 mg BID), Tac (0.5–1 mg once to twice a week), SRL (0.5–1mg once to twice a week), EVL (unknown)
Non-nucleoside reverse transcriptase inhibitors (NNRTIs)		
Delavirdine	CsA, Tac, SRL, EVL	Possible mild increase in CsA, Tac, SRL and EVL levels. TDM required
Efavirenz	CsA, Tac, SRL, EVL	Possible mild decrease in CsA, Tac, SRL and EVL levels. TDM required
Nevirapine	CsA, Tac, SRL, EVL	Possible mild decrease in CsA, Tac, SRL and EVL levels. TDM required
Etravirine	CsA, Tac, SRL, EVL	Possible alterations in CsA, Tac, SRL and EVL levels. TDM required

AZT, zidovudine/azidothymidine; Aza, azathioprine; BID, twice daily; CsA, cyclosporine A; CYP 450 cytochrome P450; Tac, tacrolimus; EVL, everolimus; MMF, mycophenolate mofetil; PI, protease inhibitor; SRL, sirolimus; TDM, therapeutic drug monitoring.

Internet references: General reference: http://medicine.iupui.edu/clinpharm/ddis/; Flockhart DA. *Drug Interactions: Cytochrome P450 Drug Interaction Table*, Indiana University School of Medicine (2007), http://medicine.iupui.edu/clinpharm/ddis/table.asp; HAART: http://www.hiv-druginteractions.org/; Micromedex® Healthcare Series [internet database], Thomson Healthcare, Greenwood Village, CO (updated periodically).

References: [1] *AST Guidelines* 2009; 9(s4): S263; [2] *Circulation* 2005; 111: 230; [3] *J HIV Therapy* 2007; 1: 24; [4] *Semin Liv Dis* 2006; 26: 273; [5] *Pharmacotherapy* 2006; 26(12): 1730; [6] *Am J Transplantation* 2007; 7: 2816; [7] Current Opinion in Nephrology and Hypertension 2009; 18: 404.

54 Antiviral Agents for Adult Transplant Recipients

Valentina Stosor

Antiviral agent	Dose	Side-effects and drug interactions	Renal and other dose adjustments
Acyclovir (Zovirax)	*IV preparation:* HSV encephalitis: 10–12.5 mg/kg q8h HSV severe mucocutaneous disease, visceral, or disseminated disease: 5–12.5 mg/kg q8h Disseminated or severe VZV: 10–12.5 mg/kg q8h *Oral preparation:* HSV mucocutanous disease (limited): 400 mg TID × 5 to 10 days HSV prophylaxis/suppression: 400–800 mg BID VZV, Shingles (limited disease): 800 mg five times/day	Irritation at IV site/phlebitis, nausea and vomiting, reversible nephrotoxocity (crystalluria) (5%), neurotoxicity (1–4%), anemia and neutropenia, elevated transaminases, pruritis, rash, headache, hematuria, hypotension	Dose based on actual body weight *Intravenous preparation:* CrCl 25–50 mL/min: 100% dose q12h CrCl 10–25 mL/min: 100% dose q24h CrCl < 10 mL/min: 50% dose q24h HD: 50% dose q24h, administer 60–100% dose after HD *Oral preparation:* CrCl 10–25 mL/min: up to 800 mg TID CrCl <10 mL/min: up to 800 mg BID HD: 200 mg BID with 400 mg after HD
Adefovir (Hepsera)	Hepatitis B: 10 mg PO q24h	Asthenia, nephrotoxocity, abdominal pain, nausea and vomiting, diarrhea, Fanconi's syndrome, lactic acidosis	CrCl 30–49 mL/min: 10 mg q48h GFR 10–29 mL/min: 10 mg q72h GFR < 10, no data HD: 10 mg every 7 d after HD
Amantadine (Symmetrel)	Influenza A treatment: 100 mg PO BID Influenza A post-exposure prophylaxis: 100 mg PO BID × 10 days after known exposure	Neurotoxicity (5–33%)[a], gastrointestinal upset	200 mg/day loading dose on first day followed by: CrCl 30–50 mL/min: 100 mg q24h CrCl 15–29 mL/min: 100 mg q48h CrCl < 15 mL/min: 100 mg qwk
Cidofovir (Vistide)	CMV induction: 5mg/kg IV wkly × two doses CMV maintenance: 5mg/kg IV q2wk With IV therapy, administer with probenecid 2g given 3 hours prior to cidofovir and 1g given 2 and 8 hours after infusion to block tubular secretion of cidofovir. Prehydrate with >1 L NS immediately before cidofovir infusion Polyomavirus-associated nephropathy: 0.25–1 mg/kg IV q1–3 weeks without probenecid	Nephrotoxicity, proteinuria, glycosuria, metabolic acidosis, Fanconi's syndrome, neutropenia (24%) Co-administration with probenecid: fever, nausea and emesis, diarrhea, headache, rash, iritis, uveitis and ocular hypotony, asthenia	The use of cidofovir is not recommended for serum creatinine >1.5 mg/dL, GFR <55 mL/min, or 2+ proteinuria, except with low doses for polyomavirus nephropathy Dose adjustments for changes in serum Cr when used for CMV treatment: Increase in serum Cr to 0.3–0.4 mg/dL above baseline: maintenance 3 mg/kg IV q2wk (with probenecid and IV hydration) Increase in SCr level to ≥0.5 above baseline or development of grade 3+ proteinuria: consider discontinue use

(Continued)

The AST Handbook of Transplant Infections, 1st edition. Edited by D. Kumar & A. Humar. © 2011 Blackwell Publishing Ltd.

Antiviral agent	Dose	Side-effects and drug interactions	Renal and other dose adjustments
Entecavir (Baraclude)	Naïve: 0.5 mg PO q24h Lamivudine-resistant HBV: 1 mg PO q24h	Generally well-tolerated, headache, fatigue, gastrointestinal intolerance, insomnia, lactic acidosis (theoretical risk)	*HBV treatment-naïve:* CrCl 30–49: 0.25 mg q24h or 0.5 mg q48h CrCl 10–29 mL/min: 0.15 mg q24h or 0.5 mg q72h CrCl < 10 mL/min; HD; or CAPD 0.05 mg q24h or 0.5 mg q7d given after HD *Lamivudine-resistant HBV:* CrCl 30–49: 0.5 mg q24h or 1 mg q48h CrCl 10–29 mL/min: 0.3 mg q24h or 1 mg q72h CrCl < 10 mL/min; HD; or CAPD: 0.1 mg q24h or 1 mg q7d
Famciclovir (Famvir)	Dermatomal zoster: 500 mg PO TID HSV mucocutaneous disease (limited): 500 mg PO BID HSV suppression/prophylaxis: 250–500 mg PO BID	Headache, nausea, diarrhea, fatigue, rash, neurotoxicity, neutropenia, abnormal liver enzyme tests	Dose adjustment for 500 mg TID is as follows: CrCl 40–59 mL/min: 500 mg q12h CrCl 20–39 mL/min: 250 mg q12h CrCl < 20 mL/min: 250 mg q24h Hemodialysis: 250 mg after each HD
Foscarnet (Foscavir)	CMV treatment: 60 mg/kg q8h or 90 mg/kg q12h for 14–21 days CMV maintenance/suppression: 90–120 mg/kg q24h Acyclovir resistant HSV or VZV: 80–120 mg/kg/day in two to three divided doses	Nephrotoxicity (33%), proteinuria, renal tubular acidosis, nephrogenic diabetes insipidus, hypocalcemia (15–35%), hypomagnesemia (15–44%), hypokalemia (10–16%), hypercalcemia, hypophosphatemia, hyperphosphatemia, neurotoxicity, fever, rash, diarrhea (30%), nausea and emesis (up to 50%), abnormal liver enzyme tests, anemia (up to 50%)	*Treatment of CMV:* CrCL 1.0–1.4 mL/min/kg: 45 mg/kg q8h CrCl 0.8–1.0 mL/min/kg: 50 mg/kg q12h CrCl 0.6–0.8 mL/min/kg: 40 mg/kg q12h CrCl 0.5–0.6 mL/min/kg: 60 mg/kg q24h CrCl 0.4–0.5 mL/min/kg: 50 mg q24h CrCl < 0.4 mL/min/kg: not recommended HD: highly removed (up to 38% with high flux filter) 50 mg/kg/dose post-HD produces serum concentrations similar to 90 mg/kg twice daily with normal renal function CVVH: use dosing for CrCl 10–50 mL/min *Maintenance for CMV:* CrCL 1.0–1.4 mL/min/kg: 90 mg/kg q24h CrCl 0.8–1.0 mL/min/kg: 65 mg/kg q24h CrCl 0.6–0.8 mL/min/kg: 105 mg/kg q48h CrCl 0.5–0.6 mL/min/kg: 80 mg/kg q48h CrCl 0.4–0.5 mL/min/kg: 65 mg/kg q48h CrCl < 0.4 mL/min/kg: not recommended

(Continued)

(Continued)

Antiviral agent	Dose	Side-effects and drug interactions	Renal and other dose adjustments
Ganciclovir (Cytovene)	*IV preparation:* CMV treatment: 5 mg/kg IV BID CMV prophylaxis or maintenance: 5 mg/kg IV q24h *Oral preparation:* CMV prophylaxis: 1 g PO TID	Neutropenia (25), thrombocytopenia (15–20%), neurotoxicity, fever, rash, hepatoxicity, phlebitis with IV infusion, nephrotoxicity	*CMV induction:* CrCl 50–69 mL/min: 2.5 mg/kg q12h CrCl 25–49 mL/min: 2.5 mg/kg q24h CrCl 10–24 mL/min: 1.25 mg/kg q24h CrCl < 10 mL/min: 1.25 mg/kg IV three times per week Hemodialysis: 1.25 mg/kg IV three times per wk following HD *CMV prophylaxis or maintenance:* CrCl 50–69 mL/min: 2.5 mg/kg q24h CrCl 25–49 mL/min: 1.25 mg/kg q24h CrCl 10–24 mL/min: 0.625 mg/kg q24h CrCl < 10 mL/min: 0.625 mg/kg IV three times per week Hemodialysis: 0.625 mg/kg IV three times per week following HD
Imiquimod (Aldara)	Apply 5% cream topically to condyloma acuminata three times weekly up to 16 weeks; wash off at 6–10 hours after application	Local reactions: erythema, irritation, pruritis, burning, tenderness, scabbing, scarring	No renal dose adjustments
Interferon-alfa-2b (Intron A)	Chronic hepatitis B: 5 MIU SC/IM q24h or 10 MIU three times weekly for 16 weeks Chronic hepatitis C: 3 MIU SC/IM three times weekly for 16 weeks; if normalization of ALT occurs at 16 weeks continue for total of 18–24 months, otherwise consider discontinuation Condyloma acuminata: 1 MU/0.1 mL injected intralesionally in up to five warts three times weekly × 3 weeks; may administer a second course at 12–16 weeks	Acute influenza-like illness, cytopenia, neuropsychiatric disturbances, thyroid abnormalities, cardiac toxicity, immune-mediated and auto-immune disorders, alopecia, nephrotoxicity, hepatotoxicity, fatigue, depression (severe in some cases)	No renal dose adjustments
Pegylated interferon-alfa-2a (Pegasys)	Chronic hepatitis B: 180 μg SC qwk × 48 weeks Chronic hepatitis C, interferon naive: 180 μg SC qwk ± ribavirin 800–1200 mg daily dose based on genotype and duration of combination therapy based on genotype Chronic hepatitis C with HIV co-infection: 180 μg SC qwk ± 800 mg ribavirin PO daily in 2 divided doses; treat for 48 wk, regardless of genotype	Same as for interferon-alfa-2b	No renal dose adjustments For ANC < 750: reduce to 135 μg qwk For platelet < 50 000: reduce to 90 μg qwk For ANC < 500 or platelet < 25 000: discontinue use

(Continued)

Antiviral agent	Dose	Side-effects and drug interactions	Renal and other dose adjustments
Pegylated interferon-alfa-2b (Peg-Intron)	Chronic hepatitis C: 1.5 μg /kg SC qwk $\pm$ ribavirin 800−1200 mg daily dose based on genotype and duration of combination therapy based on genotype	Same as for interferon-alfa-2b	No renal dose adjustments For ANC < 750 cells/mm^3 or platelets <80 000: reduce to 0.5 μg /kg. For ANC <500 or platelets <50 000: discontinue use
Lamivudine (Epivir)	Hepatitis B: 100 mg q24h	Generally well tolerated, elevated liver enzymes (with treatment of hepatitis B)	CrCl 30−49 mL/min: 100 mg first dose, then 50 mg q24h CrCl 15−29 mL/min: 35 mg first dose, then 25 mg q24h CrCl 5−14 mL/min: 35 mg first dose, then 15 mg q24h. CrCl <5 mL/min: 35 mg first dose, then 10 mg q24h
Oseltamivir (Tamiflu)	Influenza treatment: 75 mg PO BID × 5−10 days Influenza prophylaxis: 75 mg PO q24h × 10 days for post-exposure or longer for seasonal protection	Gastrointestinal upset (up to 15%), rashes, hypersensitivity reactions, hepatotoxicity, neurotoxicity	CrCl <30 mL/min: 75 mg q24h for treatment or 75 mg q48h for prophylaxis Hemodialysis: 30 mg after each HD session CAPD: 30 mg weekly
Peramivir	Influenza treatment: 600 mg IV q24h × 5−10 days	Gasrointestinal intolerance, neutropenia, neuropsychiatric disturbances, hyperglycemia, rash	CrCl 31−49 mL/min: 150 mg q24h CrCl 10−30 mL/min: 100 mg q24h CrCl < 10 mL/min: 100mg on day 1 then 15 mg q24h Hemodialysis: 100 mg on day 1 then 100 mg 2 hours after each HD session on HD days Peritoneal dialysis: no recommendations
Podofilox (Condylox)	Condyloma acuminata: apply 5% solution or gel to warts BID for 3 days followed by 4 days of no therapy; may repeat weekly up to four cycles. Daily application not to exceed 10 cm/m^2	Local reactions, gastrointestinal upset, confusion, thrombocytopenia, areflexia	No renal dose adjustments
Ribavirin (Rebetrol, Virazole)	Oral preparation for hepatitis C infection: >75 kg: 1200 mg PO q24h <75 kg: 1000 mg PO q24h <40 kg: 800 mg PO q24h Aerosol preparation (for respiratory syncytial virus): reservoir concentration 20 mg/mL administered over 18 hours once daily or 60 mg/mL administered over 2 hours TID	*Oral preparation:* Hemolytic anemia, respiratory symptoms, pruritis, myalgia, rash, nausea, depression, nervousness, anorexia, insomnia, lactic acidosis, *Aerosolized preparation:*[b] Conjunctival irritation, bronchospasm, acute water intoxication	CrCl < 50: not recommended; consider dose reduction CrCl < 10 mL/min: not recommended. Consider dose reduction Hemodialysis: not recommended; consider dose reduction. Administer dose after HD

(Continued)

(Continued)

Antiviral agent	Dose	Side-effects and drug interactions	Renal and other dose adjustments
Rimantadine (Flumadine)	Influenza treatment: 100 mg PO BID Influenza prophylaxis: 100 mg PO BID	Neurotoxicity, gastrointestinal upset (co-administration with TMP-SMX may result in increased neurotoxicity)	CrCl <10 mL/min: 100 mg q24h Severe hepatic dysfunction: 100 mg q24h For age ≥65 years: 100 mg q24h
Trifluridine (Viroptic)	HSV keratoconjuctivitis: 1 gtt of 1% solution q2h, up to 9 gtts q24h	Ocular discomfort, palpebral edema, hypersensitivity reactions	No renal dose adjustments
Valacyclovir (Valtrex)	Mucocutaneous HSV (limited): 1 g PO BID HSV suppression/prophylaxis: 500 mg PO BID Dermatomal zoster (limited): 1 g PO TID	Headache, gastrointestinal upset, thrombotic microangiopathy	CrCl 30–49 mL/min: 1 g BID CrCl 10–29 mL/min: 1 g q24h CrCl < 10 mL/min: 500 mg q24h
Valganciclovir[c] (Valcyte)	CMV treatment: 900 mg PO BID CMV prophylaxis or maintenance: 900 mg PO q24h	Leukopenia (see 'Ganciclovir' for other side-effects)	*CMV treatment:* CrCl 40–59 mL/min: 450 mg BID CrCl 25–39 mL/min: 450 mg q24h CrCl 10–24 mL/min: 450 mg q48h CrCl <10 mL/min: not recommended Hemodialysis: not recommended *CMV prophylaxis or maintenance:* CrCl 40–59 mL/min: 450 mg q24h CrCl 25–39 mL/min: 450 mg q48h CrCl 10–24 mL/min: 450 mg 2x per wk CrCl <10 mL/min: not recommended Hemodialysis: not recommended
Zanamavir (Relenza)	10 mg BID by inhaler	Bronchospasm	No renal dose adjustments

ALT, alanine transaminase; ANC, absolute neutrophil count; BID, twice daily; CAPD, continuous ambulatory peritoneal dialysis; CrCl, creatinine clearance; CMV, cytomegalovirus; CVVH, continuous veno-venous hemofiltration; GFR, glomerular filtration rate; HBV, hepatitis B virus; HD, hemodialysis; IV, intravenous; NS, normal saline; PO, by mouth; SC, subcutaneous; TID, three times a day; TMP-SMX, trimethoprim-sulfamethoxazole; VZV, varicella zoster virus.

[a]Co-administration with TMP-SMX may result in increased neurotoxicity.

[b]Aerosolized ribavirin use is limited by lack of/inconsistent efficacy, occupational exposure risks, difficulty of administration, and cost.

[c]Valganciclovir is not approved by the US FDA for use in liver transplant recipients.

References: [1] *Am J Transplantation* 2009; 9(s4): S136; [2] *Am J Transplantation* 2009; 9(s4): S166; [3] *Hepatology* 2009; 50: 1; [4] *Am J Transplantation* 2009; 9(s4): S108; [5] *Am J Transplantation* 2009; 9(s4): S104; [6] Hayden FG (2005). Antiviral agents (other than antiretrovirals). In: Mandell GL, Bennett JE, Dolin R, eds. *Principles and Practice of Infectious Diseases*, 6th edn, Elsevier, Philadelphia PA, p. 514.

55   Antifungal Agents in Adult Transplant Recipients

Shmuel Shoham

Triazoles

Agent; how supplied	Common clinical uses	Loading dose	Dosage (IV)	Dosage (oral)	Adjustment for decreased GFR	Common adverse events/ comments
Fluconazole (IV, oral suspension, tablets)	Candidiasis (mucosal, invasive and symptomatic cystitis), cryptococcosis (stable disease), coccidioidomycosis, prophylaxis	Invasive candidiasis: 800 mg Esophageal candidiasis: 400 mg	Systemic infections: 400 mg/day Oropharyngeal candidiasis: 100–200 mg/day Esophageal candidiasis: 200–400 mg/day Candida cystitis: 200 mg/day Estimated price for 400 mg: IV, $65	Systemic infections: 400 mg/day Oropharyngeal candidiasis: 100–200 mg/day Esophageal candidiasis: 200–400 mg/day Candida cystitis: 200 mg/day Estimated price for 400 mg: tablet, $3; solution, $65	Loading dose 400 mg Maintenance: CrCl < 50 mL/min, 50% dose reduction Hemodialysis: 100% of dose given after dialysis	Some *Candida* sp. are resistant to fluconazole Important drug interactions with CNI and mTOR inhibitors Rare cases of severe liver toxicity Rare allergic reactions with anaphylaxis and dermatitis Alopecia with long term use QT interval prolongation
Itraconazole (IV, oral solution, capsules)	Aspergillosis (stable disease), histoplasmosis (stable disease), blastomycosis, refractory mucosal candidiasis, prophylaxis, empirical therapy in febrile neutropenia	IV: 200 mg BID × 4 doses PO: 200 mg TID × 3 days	Systemic infection: 200 mg once daily to BID Estimated price for 200 mg: IV, $200	Systemic infection: 200 mg once daily to BID Prophylaxis: 200 mg/day Empiric therapy: 200 mg BID Oropharyngeal or esophageal candidiasis: 200 mg/day Estimated price for 200 mg: capsule, $14; solution, $18	PO: limited data, but consider using 50% of dose with CrCl <10 mL/min IV: concern about accumulation of carrier molecule (cyclodextrin) in patients with reduced CrCl	Avoid in patients with history of CHF Rare cases of severe liver toxicity, CHF Measure blood levels of itraconazole after 2 weeks to ensure effective levels. Bioavailability improves with oral solution or acidic beverages if using tablets Itraconazole is a potent CYP3A4 inhibitor,

Drug	Spectrum/Indications	Dose	Dose adjustment	Comments/Side-effects
Voriconazole (IV, oral suspension, tablets)	Invasive aspergillosis, systemic and refractory mucosal candidiasis, fusariosis, scedosporiosis, prophylaxis	IV: 6 mg/kg q12h for 1 day; Filamentous infections: 4 mg/kg BID; Invasive candidiasis: 3–4 mg/kg BID; Estimated price for 200 mg: IV, $90; >40 kg adults: 200 mg BID; <40 kg adults: 100 mg BID; Inadequate response to oral therapy: increase dose by 50%; Estimated price for 200 mg: tablet, $30; suspension, $40;	PO: no dose adjustment; IV: concern about accumulation of carrier molecule (cyclodextrin) in patients with reduced CrCl	with potential for life-threatening drug interactions including with CNI and mTOR inhibitors; GI side-effects are common, especially with cyclodextrin solution; QT interval prolongation; Therapeutic drug monitoring may be helpful as levels vary between individuals (e.g. slow metabolizers due to isoenzyme polymorphisms); Visual disturbances, hallucinations, photosensitivity rash, liver toxicity; Voriconazole has multiple and complex effects on CYP enzymes and potential for life-threatening drug interactions, including with CNI and mTOR inhibitors; QT interval prolongation
Posaconazole (oral suspension)	Prophylaxis in AML and GVHD, refractory mucosal candidiasis, refractory aspergillosis, Zygomyces infections, other refractory mould infections	None; Prophylaxis: 200 mg TID; Therapy: 400 mg BID; Estimated price for 200 mg: suspension, $30	None	Several days are required for the drug to reach steady-state levels; Bioavailability improved with high-fat meals; GI side-effects common; Posaconazole is a CYP3A4 inhibitor with potential for life-threatening drug interactions, including with CNI and mTOR inhibitors; QT interval prolongation

(Continued)

147

Agent; how supplied	Common clinical uses	Loading dose	Dosage (IV)	Dosage (oral)	Adjustment for decreased GFR	Common adverse events/ comments
Echinocandins						
Caspofungin (IV)	Invasive candidiasis, refractory mucosal candidiasis, empirical therapy in neutropenia and fever, invasive aspergillosis, micafungin indicated for prophylaxis in HSCT	70 mg	50 mg/day
Estimated price for 50 mg: $200–300	None	None	Rare: allergic reactions, histamine release, liver function abnormalities, pain at site of infusion
Micafungin (IV)	As caspofungin	None	50–150 mg/day
Estimated price for 100 mg: $100–200	None	None	As caspofungin
Anidulafungin (IV)	As caspofungin	200 mg	100 mg/day	None	None	As caspofungin
Polyenes						
Amphotericin B deoxycholate (IV, aerosolized)	Cryptococcosis, histoplasmosis, invasive zygomyces, empirical therapy in neutropenia and fever, invasive aspergillosis, invasive candidiasis (including CNS disease), rare filamentous fungal infections	None	Systemic infection: 0.7–1 mg/kg/day
Aerosolized: 10–20 mg once daily to BID
Estimated price for 50 mg: $12	None	None	Major renal, electrolyte, and infusion-related toxicity
Not commonly used in transplant patients due to nephrotoxicity
Aerosolized amphotericin may be used for prophylaxis in lung transplant patients, but monitor for bronchospasm

Lipid formulation Amphotericin B (IV, aerosolized) (ABLC or Ambisome)	As amphotericin B deoxycholate	None	Systemic infection: 3–5 mg/kg/day Empirical therapy: 3 mg/kg/day Estimated price for 350 mg: $800–1,300	None	Reduced renal and electrolyte toxicity relative to dAmB Aerosolized lipid formulations have been used in varying doses for prophylaxis in lung transplant patients
Other					
Flucytosine (oral capsule)	Combination therapy for CNS cryptococcosis and CNS candidiasis Not for use as monotherapy	None	25–37.5 mg/kg QID Estimated price for 500 mg capsule: $10	Use with extreme caution in renal impairment: CrCl 20–40 mL/min: dose BID CrCl 10–19 mL/min: dose once daily CrCl <10 mL/min: avoid if possible	Bone marrow and hepatic toxicity especially with decreased CrCl Measure drug levels to reduce chance of toxicity

ABLC, amphotericin B lipid complex; AML, acute myeloid leukemia; BID, twice daily; CHF, congestive heart failure; CNI, calcineurin inhibitor; CNS, central nervous system; CrCl, creatinine clearance; CYP, cytochrome P450; dAmB, amphotericin B deoxycholate ; GFR, glomerular filtration rate; GI, gastrointestinal; GVHD, graft-versus-host disease; HSCT, hematopoietic stem cell transplant; IV, intravenous; mTOR, mammalian target of rapamycin; PO, by mouth; TID, three times a day.

The AST Handbook of Transplant Infections, 1st edition. Edited by D. Kumar & A. Humar. © 2011 Blackwell Publishing Ltd.

56 Antiviral Agents for Pediatric Transplant Recipients

Lara Danziger-Isakov, Lizbeth Hansen & Elizabeth Neuner

Antiviral/indications	Dosing		Renal impairment	Interacting drug	Effect	Comment
	Treatment	Prophylaxis				
Acyclovir						
HSV (cutaneous)						
<12 years	IV: 10 mg/kg/dose q8h *Alternative:* 250 mg/m²/dose q8h		CrCl 25–50 mL/min: normal dose q12h CrCl 10–25 mL/min: normal dose q24h CrCl < 10 mL/min: 50% of dose q24h	Mycophenolate	May increase serum concentration of acyclovir in the presence of renal impairment	BSA-based dosing: 500 mg/m² = 20 mg/kg 250 mg/m² = 10 mg/kg Use Ideal body weight (IBW) for dosing in obese patients
	PO: 80 mg/kg/day in three to five divided doses (not to exceed 1 g/day)	PO: 600–1000 mg/day in three to five divided doses	–	Concurrent nephrotoxins (e.g. aminoglycosides, amphotericin)	Increased risk of nephrotoxicity. Ensure adequate hydration; monitor renal function	Some centers have used up to 2 g/day of oral acyclovir in children < 12 years
≥12 years	IV: 5 mg/kg/dose q8h PO: 400 mg five times/day	PO: 600–1000 mg/day in three to five divided doses	–	–	–	–
HSV (encephalitis)						
<12 years	IV: 20 mg/kg/dose q8h Alternative: 500 mg/m²/dose q8h		CrCl 25–50 mL/min: normal dose q12h CrCl 10–25 mL/min: normal dose q24h CrCl <10 mL/min: 50% of dose q24h	–	–	–

≥12 years	IV: 10–15 mg/kg/dose q8h	—	CrCl 25–50 mL/min: normal dose q12h CrCl 10–25 mL/min: normal dose q24h CrCl <10 mL/min: 50% of dose q24h	—
Varicella zoster virus				
<12 years	IV: 20 mg/kg/dose q8h	—	CrCl 25–50 mL/min: normal dose q12h CrCl 10–25 mL/min: normal dose q24h CrCl <10 mL/min: 50% of dose q24h	—
≥12 years	IV: 10 mg/kg/dose q8h	—	CrCl 25–50 mL/min: normal dose q12h CrCl 10–25 mL/min: normal dose q24h CrCl <10 mL/min: 50% of dose q24h	—
Ganciclovir				
CMV	*Induction V:* 15 mg/kg/dose q12h	*Maintenance* IV: 5 mg/kg/dose q24h	*Induction:* CrCl 50–69 mL/min: 2.5 mg/kg q12h CrCl 25–49 mL/min: 2.5 mg/kg q24h	Imipenem	May enhance the adverse effect (seizures) of imipenem Risk versus benefit ratio should be considered	—
			CrCl 10–24 mL/min: 1.25 mg/kg q24h CrCl <10 mL/min 1.25 mg/kg/dose three times per week following hemodialysis	Probenecid	Increases concentrations of ganciclovir	

(Continued)

151

(Continued)

Antiviral/indications	Dosing		Renal impairment	Interacting drug	Effect	Comment
	Treatment	Prophylaxis				
			Maintenance: CrCl 50–69 mL/min: 2.5 mg/kg q24 h CrCl 25–49 mL/min: 1.25 mg/kg q24 h CrCl 10–24 mL/min: 0.625 mg/kg q24	Mycophenolate	Increased marrow toxicity	
			CrCl < 10 mL/min 0.625 mg/kg/dose three times per week following hemodialysis	Concurrent nephrotoxins (e.g. amioglycosides, amphotericin etc.)	Increased risk of nephrotoxicity	
Valganciclovir *CMV* ≥18 years old	*Induction* PO: 18–20 mg/kg/ dose q12 h (not to exceed 900 mg/ dose)	*Maintenance* PO: 18–20 mg/kg/ dose once daily (not to exceed 900 mg/dose)	*Induction:* CrCl 40–59 mL/min: 50% of dose q12 h CrCl 25–39 mL/min: 50% of dose q24 h CrCl 10–24 mL/min: 50% of dose QOD CrCl <10 mL/min: 50% of dose following hemodialysis (limited data available) *Maintenance:* CrCl 40–59 mL/min: 50% of dose q24 h CrCl 25–39 mL/min: 50% of dose QOD CrCl 10–24 mL/min: 50% of dose twice weekly CrCl <10 mL/min: 50% of dose following hemodialysis (limited data available)	See 'Ganciclovir' interactions	–	–

4 months to 16 years old (new manufacturer labeling)	PO: (7 × body surface area × CrCl) once daily (not to exceed 900 mg/dose)	Dosing calculation accounts for renal dysfunction	—	—	—
Amantadine *Influenza A*					
1–9 years or >10 years *and* <40 kg	PO: 5 mg/kg/day in one to two divided doses (not to exceed 150 mg/day)	CrCl 30–50 mL/min: full dose on day 1, then decrease to 50% of dose thereafter	Anticholinergic agents (belladonna, benztropine, etc.)	May enhance anticholinergic adverse effects	Check local/national guidelines based on influenza resistance patterns before use
		CrCl 15–29 mL/min: full dose on day 1, then decrease to 50% of dose given every other day	Antipsychotic agents (thioridazine, etc.)	May enhance anticholinergic adverse effects	
		CrCl <15 mL/min: full dose given every 7 days	Trimethoprim	May enhance the CNS toxicity (including delirum or myoclonus) of amantadine	
>10 years or >40 kg	PO: 100 mg BID PO: 100 mg BID	CrCl 30–50 mL/min: full dose on day 1, then decrease to 50% of dose thereafter	—	—	—
		CrCl 15–29 mL/min: full dose on day 1, then decrease to 50% of dose given every other day			
		CrCl < 15 mL/min: full dose given every 7 days			

(Continued)

Antiviral/indications	Dosing		Renal impairment	Interacting drug	Effect	Comment
	Treatment	Prophylaxis				
Rimantadine						
Influenza A						
1–9 years or >10 years *and* <40 kg	PO: 5 mg/kg/day in one to two divided doses (not to exceed 150 mg/day)	PO: 5 mg/kg/day in one to two divided doses (not to exceed 150 mg/day)	No adjustment for CrCl >10 mL/min CrCl ≤ 10 mL/min: 50% dose decrease	See 'Amantadine' interactions	–	Check local/national guidelines based on influenza resistance patterns before use
>10 years or >40 kg	PO: (adult dosing) 100 mg BID	PO: (adult dosing) 100 mg BID	No adjustment for CrCl >10 mL/min CrCl ≤10 mL/min: 50% dose decrease	–	–	Has fewer CNS toxicities than amantadine
Oseltamivir						
Influenza A & B						
<3 months	PO: 12 mg BID for 5 days	Not recommended unless situation is judged critical due to limited data in this age group	CrCl 10–30 mL/min: *treatment* – normal dose once daily; *prophylaxis* – normal dose every other day	–	–	Check local/national guidelines based on influenza resistance patterns before use
3–5 months	PO: 20 mg BID for 5 days	PO: 20 mg once daily for 10 days	CrCl 10–30 mL/min: *treatment* – normal dose once daily; *prophylaxis* – normal dose every other day	–	–	–
6–11 months	PO: 25 mg BID for 5 days	PO: 25 mg once daily for 10 days	CrCl 10–30 mL/min: *treatment* – normal dose once daily; *prophylaxis* – normal dose every other day	–	–	–

	Treatment	Prophylaxis	Renal/hepatic adjustment		Comments
≥12 months *and* ≤15kg	PO: 30mg BID for 5 days	PO: 30mg once daily for 10 days	CrCl 10–30mL/min: *treatment* – normal dose once daily; *prophylaxis* – normal dose every other day	–	–
≥12 months *and* >15kg and <23kg	PO: 45mg BID for 5 days	PO: 45mg once daily for 10 days	CrCl 10–30mL/min: *treatment* – normal dose once daily; *prophylaxis* – normal dose every other day	–	–
>12 months AND ≥23 to <40kg	PO: 60mg BID for 5 days	PO: 60mg once daily for 10 days	CrCl 10–30mL/min: *treatment* – normal dose once daily; *prophylaxis* – normal dose every other day	–	–
≥12 months AND ≥40kg	PO: 75mg BID for 5 days	PO: 75mg once daily for 10 days	CrCl 10–30mL/min: *treatment* – normal dose once daily; *prophylaxis* – normal dose every other day	–	–

Zanamivir

Influenza A and B

	Treatment	Prophylaxis	Renal/hepatic adjustment		Comments
Children ≥5 years		INH: 10mg once daily for 10 days	No renal or hepatic adjustment	–	Check local/national guidelines based on influenza resistance patterns before use
Children ≥7 years and adults	INH: 10mg twice daily (12 hours apart) for 5 days	INH: 10mg once daily for 10 days	–	–	Inhalation powder not to be solubilized and administered via nebulizer or mechanical ventilator

(Continued)

Antiviral/indications	Dosing		Renal impairment	Interacting drug	Effect	Comment
	Treatment	Prophylaxis				
Ribavirin						
RSV	NEB: 20 mg/mL (6 g reconstituted with 300 mL of sterile water without preservatives). Aerosolized over 12–18 hours/day. Use with Viratek® small particle aerosol generator (SPAG-2)		Unknown if renal adjustment is needed for inhalation. Oral tablets are contraindicated if CrCl <50 ml/min	Azathioprine	Increased risk of azathioprine-induced myelotoxicity; decreased active 6-TH metabolites	Requires a negative pressure room and additional precautions for healthcare workers. Caution with use in mechanical ventilation
Palivizumab						
RSV	Limited data available	IM: 15 mg/kg once monthly during RSV season (for cardiopulmonary bypass patients, administer a dose as soon as possible after cardiopulmonary bypass procedure, even if <1 month from previous dose)	No renal or hepatic adjustment	–	–	–
<2 years old and meets criteria for prophylaxis						
Foscarnet						
Resistant CMV OR CMV (retinitis)	*Induction* IV: 180 mg/kg/day divided q8h for 14–21 days. *Maintenance* IV: 90–120 mg/kg/ day as a single daily dose		Renal adjustment varies with indication. Please refer to package insert for renal dosing	Concurrent nephrotoxins (e.g. amioglycosides, amphotericin)	Increased risk of nephrotoxicity	Monitor for electrolyte imbalances, including hypocalemia, hypo- or hyperphosphatemia, hypokalemia or hypomagnesemia

		Induction	Maintenance	Monitoring	Drug interactions	
					QTc prolonging agents (e.g. fluoroquinolones, methadone, azole antifungals)	Increased risk for QTc prolongation
					Medications that lower seizure threshold (e.g. imipenem, fluoroquinolones)	May increase risk of seizures due to electrolyte imbalance caused by foscarnet
					Pentamidine	Increased risk of hypocalcemia
Cidofovir						
	CMV (retinitis)	IV: 5 mg/kg/dose × 1 dose with probenecid and hydration[a]	IV: 5 mg/kg/dose every other week with probenecid and hydration[a]	If creatinine rises > 0.3–0.4 mg/dL: 3 mg/kg/dose weekly If creatinine rises ≥0.5 mg/dL or development of ≥ 3+ proteinuria: consider discontinue therapy	Concurrent nephrotoxins (e.g. aminoglycosides, amphotericin)	Increased risk of nephrotoxicity. Ensure adequate hydration[a]
	Adenovirus	(Limited data available) IV: 5 mg/kg/dose once weekly Alternative: 3 mg/kg/dose once weekly Alternative: 1 mg/kg/dose three times a week with probenecid and hydration[a]	–	–	–	

6-TH, 6-Thioguanine; BID, twice daily; BSA, body surface area; CMV, cytomegalovirus; CNI, calcineurin inhibitor; CNS, central nervous system; CrCl, creatinine clearance; HSV, herpes simplex virus; IM, intramuscular; INH, isoniazid; IV, intravenous; NEB, nebulization; PO, by mouth; QOD, every other day; RSV, respiratory syncytial virus.

[a]Probenecid – PO: 1.25 g/m² given 3 hours prior, 1 hour after and 8 hours after cidofovir infusion. Hydration – IV: normal saline bolus equal to three times maintenance administered 1 hour and 1 hour after cidofovir infusion, then decrease to two times maintenance for the subsequent 2 hours.

The AST Handbook of Transplant Infections, 1st edition. Edited by D. Kumar & A. Humar. © 2011 Blackwell Publishing Ltd.

57 Antifungal Agents for Pediatric Transplant Recipients

Lara Danziger-Isakov, Lizbeth Hansen & Elizabeth Neuner

Antifungals class	Indications	Dosing (treatment unless noted otherwise)	Renal or hepatic dosing	Interacting drug[a] and effect	Comments
Triazoles					
Itraconazole	Histoplasmosis, blastomycosis, coccidiodomycosis (non-severe or convalescence) Severe blastomycosis	PO: 5–10 mg/kg/day in two divided doses (not to exceed 400 mg/day) IV: 2.5–5 mg/kg/day	No renal or hepatic adjustment	*Antacids* (magnesium, aluminum, calcium containing): decrease absorption of itraconazole; give antacids 1 hour before or 2 hours after itraconazole *Benzodiazepines*: contraindicated with alprazolam, oral midazolam, and triazolam. Increased levels/effects of benzodiazepines *Calcium-channel blockers*: increased CCB levels and risk of adverse effects *Cisapride*: contraindicated; increased risk of QTc prolongation due to decreased cisapride metabolism *Cyclosporine*: increased cyclosporine levels; some centers recommend 50–75% cyclosporine dose reduction *H₂ antagonists*: reduced itraconazole absorption *HMG-CoA reductase inhibitors*: contraindicated with lovastatin and simvastatin; increased risk of skeletal muscle toxicity *Phenytoin*: avoid combination; significantly decreases levels of itraconazole *Proton pump inhibitors*: avoid combination; reduced itraconazole absorption *Quinidine*: contraindicated; increased risk of quinidine toxicity	Capsule and oral solution are not bioequivalent. Capsule should be taken with food. Solution should be taken on an empty stomach Caution in history of ventricular dysfunction or CHF

Voriconazole	Aspergillus, Scedosporium, Fusarium				
		< 12 years	Treatment (IDSA guidelines): IV: 7 mg/kg/dose every 12 hours PO (limited data available): 7 mg/kg/dose every 12 hours Prophylaxis (limited data available): IV, PO: 3–4 mg/kg/dose every 12 hours	CrCl < 50 mL/min: switch to PO voriconazole Mild-to-moderate hepatic dysfunction (Child–Pugh class A and B): following standard loading dose, reduce maintenance dosage by 50%	*Rifampin/rifabutin*: avoid combination; significantly decreases itraconazole levels *Sirolimus*: significantly increases sirolimus levels; dose reduction required *Tacrolimus*: significantly increases tacrolimus levels; some centers recommend 50–75% tacrolimus dose reduction *Wafarin*: increased INR and risk of bleeding. *Benzodiazepines*: caution with alprazolam and midazolam; increased levels/effect of benzodiazepines
		≥ 12 years	IV: 6 mg/kg/dose every 12 hours for 1 day then 4 mg/kg/dose every 12 hours PO (limited data available): 6mg/kg/dose every 12 hours for 1 day then 4 mg/kg/dose every 12 hours		*Calcium-channel blockers*: increased CCB levels and risk of adverse effects *Carbamazepine*: contraindicated; decreased voriconazole levels *Clarithromycin*: may increase clarithromycin levels and risk of QTc prolongation *Cyclosporine*: increased cyclosporine levels; recommend 50% cyclosporine dose reduction. Frequent monitoring required *HMG-CoA reductase inhibitors*: increased HMG-CoA reductase inhibitors levels and risk of toxicity *Methadone*: increased methadone levels and risk of toxicity; dose adjustment may be necessary *Oral hypoglycemics (glipizide, glyburide, etc.)*: avoid combination; consider dose reduction of hypoglycemics

Voriconazole absorption is increased on an empty stomach. Administer 1 hour before or 1 hour after meals

(Continued)

Antifungals class	Indications	Dosing (treatment unless noted otherwise)	Renal or hepatic dosing	Interacting drug[a] and effect	Comments
				Phenobarbital: contraindicated; significantly decreases voriconazole levels	
				Phenytoin: decreases voriconazole levels and increases phenytoin levels; dose adjustments required	
				Quinidine: contraindicated; increased risk of quinidine toxicity	
				QTc prolonging medications: contraindicated with cisapride, pimozide, or quinidine; increased risk for QTc prolongation	
				Rifampin/rifabutin: contraindicated; decreased voriconazole levels	
				Sirolimus: contraindicated; if use is unavoidable, significant dose adjustments may be required due to increased levels of sirolimus	
				St John's Wort: contraindicated; decreased voriconazole levels	
				Tacrolimus: increased tacrolimus levels and risk of toxicity; some centers recommend 75% dose decrease of tacrolimus	
				Wafarin: increased INR and risk of bleeding. Dose adjustments may be necessary.	
Fluconazole	Candidasis, cryptoccoccosis	IV, PO: 6–12 mg/kg/day (not to exceed 800 mg/day)	CrCl ≤ 50 mL/min: 50% dose	*Benzodiazepines*: increased levels of alprazolam, midazolam, and triazolam	Not appropriate empiric therapy for disseminated infection due to resistance of some strains, including *Candida krusei*
				Anti-arrhythmics (dolfetilide, sotalol, etc.): increased risk for QTc prolongation	
				Carbamazepine: increased carbamazepine levels	
				Cyclosporine: increased cyclosporine levels and risk of toxicity	
				Fluoroquinolones: increased risk for QTc prolongation	

				HMG-CoA reductase inhibitors: may increase levels and risk of toxicity of HMG-CoA reductase inhibitors
				Methadone: increased methadone levels and risk of toxicity
				Phenytoin: increased phenytoin levels
				Quinidine: not recommended; increased quinidine toxicity
				Rifabutin: increase rifabutin levels and risk of toxicity
				Rifampin: decreased fluconazole levels; dose adjustments may be required
				Sirolimus: increased sirolimus levels and risk of toxicity
				Tacrolimus: increased tacrolimus levels; monitor therapy
				Wafarin: increased INR and risk of bleeding
Posaconazole				
	< 13 years	PO (limited data available): 10–20mg/kg/day divided into two to four doses/day (not to exceed 800mg/day)	No renal or hepatic adjustment	See drug interactions for itraconazole	Posaconazole absorption is increased when given with high-fat meals
	≥ 13 years	PO: 800mg/day divided into two to four doses/day	No renal or hepatic adjustment		
Clotrimazole	Oral candidiasis ≥ 3 years	PO: 10mg troche five times per day	No renal or hepatic adjustment	*Sirolimus*: may increase sirolimus levels; monitor therapy	

(Continued)

Antifungals class	Indications	Dosing (treatment unless noted otherwise)	Renal or hepatic dosing	Interacting drug[a] and effect	Comments
				Tacrolimus: may increase tacrolimus levels; monitor therapy	
Polyenes					
Amphotericin B deoxycholate (AmB-D)	Candidiasis, *Aspergillus*, cryptococcosis (including meningitis), blastomycoses, mucormycosis, *Fusarium*	IV: 0.25–1 mg/kg/day; infuse over 2–6 hours Rapidly progressing disease may require 1.5 mg/kg/day	No renal or hepatic adjustment	Concurrent nephrotoxins (e.g. amioglycosides, ganciclovir) – increased risk of nephrotoxicity; monitor renal function	
Amphotericin B lipid complex (ABLC)	Candidiasis, *Aspergillus*, cryptococcosis (including meningitis), blastomycoses, mucormycosis, *Fusarium*	IV: 3– 5 mg/kg/day	No renal or hepatic adjustment		
Amphotericin B liposomal (L-AmB)	Candidiasis, *Aspergillus*, mucormycosis, *Fusarium*, histoplasmosis	IV: 3–5 mg/kg/day (some centers have used up to a maximum of 10 mg/kg/day)	No renal or hepatic adjustment		
	Candidal meningitis	IV: 5 mg/kg/day	No renal or hepatic adjustment		
	Cryptococcal meningitis (in HIV+)	IV: 6 mg/kg/day	No renal or hepatic adjustment		
Amphotericin B cholesteryl sulfate complex (ABCD)	*Aspergillus, Fusarium*	IV: 3–4 mg/kg/day; 6 mg/kg/day for severe infection; maximum 7.5 mg/kg/day	No renal or hepatic adjustment		

Echinocandins

Caspofungin	Candidasis and aspergillosis 3 months to 17 years	IV: 70 mg/m² on day 1; subsequent dosing 50 mg/m² once daily (not to exceed 70 mg on day 1 and 50 mg on subsequent days)	No renal adjustment; no pediatric clinical data to support hepatic adjustments	Concomitant use with enzyme inducers (rifampin, efavirenz, nevirapine, phenytoin, dexamethasone, or carbamazepine) – consider increasing dose to 70 mg/m² IV once daily Tacrolimus – decreased tacrolimus levels. Monitor closely and dose adjustments may be necessary
Anidulafungin	Candidasis	IV (limited data available):1.5 mg/kg/day (not to exceed 100 mg/ day)	No renal or hepatic adjustment	Reconstituted with a dehydrated alcohol; a 50 mg vial contains approximately 3 g of ethanol
Micafungin	Candidasis and aspergillosis	IV: 4–6 mg/kg/day IV (up to 10–12 mg/kg/ day in neonates) (not to exceed 100 mg/ day or 150 mg/day in severe infections)	No renal or hepatic adjustment	

CCB, calcium-channel blocker; CHF, congestive heart failure; CrCl, creatinine clearance; HIV, human immunodeficiency virus; HMG-CoA, 3-hydroxy-3-methylglutaryl-coenzyme A; HSV, herpes simplex virus; IDSA, Infectious Diseases Society of America; INR, international normalized ratio; IV, intravenous; PO, by mouth.

ªList is not exhaustive.

The AST Handbook of Transplant Infections, 1st edition. Edited by D. Kumar & A. Humar. © 2011 Blackwell Publishing Ltd.

Index